M
14.95

Help Yourself

Problem Solving
for the Disabled

D1252912

Douglas R. Bucy

Illustrated by
Rebecca A. Nolan

Macmillan · USA

The information contained herein is obtained from sources which I have used and believe are reliable and is included here for general information purposes only. The references and product suggestions are not intended to disseminate either medical or legal advice, and I disclaim any liability for the accuracy thereof. The reader should obtain medical or legal advice from their own physician or attorney in each instance.

Help Yourself: Problem Solving for the Disabled

Macmillan General Reference
A Simon & Schuster Macmillan Company
1633 Broadway
New York, NY 10019

Manufactured in the United States of America

1   2   3   4   5   6   7   8   9

Library of Congress Cataloging-in-Publication Data

Bucy, Douglas R., 1931-1995.
    Help yourself : problem solving for the disabled / Douglas R. Bucy
    : illustrated by Rebecca A. Nolan.
    p. cm.
    ISBN 0–02–861059-8
    1. Physically handicapped--Services for--United States.
    2. Physically handicapped--Medical care--United States.
    3. Physically handicapped--Mental health services--United States.
    I. Title.
    HV3020.2.U6B83   1996
    362.4'048'0973--dc20   96-16206
                                                      CIP

Contents

PART II • **Day-to-Day Living**

PART III • **Finding Help Within**

PART IV • **Money Matters**

Illustrations

Foreword

Acceptance is not defeat.

Courage is not being without fear, but to go forward in spite of fear.

It was with these two mottoes that Doug and I endeavored to live our lives ever since that fateful day in October 1992 when we first learned that Doug had ALS (Lou Gehrig's disease). At first it seemed unreal—a bad dream from which we would eventually awaken. But as time went on, and as we sought out neurologist after neurologist specializing in ALS, we began to come to grips with the fact that our lives would never be the same again.

During his life, Doug was driven by two axioms: "Good enough is not good enough," and "There is nothing that I can't do—or at least try." As a boy and a young man, Doug excelled at achieving his goals as he progressed through his school years. As a man, he enlisted in the Army rather than waiting to be drafted. Doug was a wonderful husband, a loving father to four daughters, and a gentle grandfather to eight grandchildren. He was an active churchman, and a businessman who lived by an unblemished code of ethics.

Early in our marriage, which began in December 1955, Doug and I discovered that we had a certain ESP with each other—one of us having a thought and the other verbalizing that exact thought, and vice versa. As you read this book you will find a reference to my being able to "read" Doug. It is my strong conviction that this extra sense helped us to be more sensitive to each other as his disease progressed.

When ALS struck, our whole family became victims. However, we were determined not to be "victimized," but to support each other throughout. We have become a stronger family as a result. Doug wrote in February of 1995: "Since we do not have any guarantee about tomorrow, we must live each day to its fullest and not waste any time with petty or insignificant things. I feel very strongly that God is giving me time and strength to help others who are depressed and beaten in this daily struggle we call life. It gives me good feelings to be able to help someone else get a different perspective on their situation."

Doug did have "down" times, and it was then that he learned to cry. It was the only outlet he had to help him vent his anger and frustration over the disease that was slowly robbing him of his life. At this time, he wrote a lovely prayer, the essence of which was "give me peace."

Doug felt that as long as he was productive, life was worth living. He continued working as long as he could as a self-employed business consultant specializing in small business management. When he could no longer continue, instead of saying "I give up," he decided to write a book—this book. Since he could no longer type, he purchased a voice-activated computer from "Voice for Joanie" with the help of our friend and the program's creator, Shirley Fredlund. Once he was set up, there was no stopping him. He talked to his computer every day.

During this time, he was also volunteering for an ALS drug study at the University of Connecticut Medical Center in Farmington, Connecticut. Doug kept a daily journal of the study up until six days before he passed away in November 1995. Although Doug did not live to see this book published, he did have the satisfaction of receiving a signed contract; he knew the book would be a reality. He was overjoyed at the prospect of being an author, an accomplishment he might not have achieved had he not been faced with ALS.

Doug was a multi-talented man. He loved working with wood; he painted landscapes in oil. When he could no longer hold the paintbrush in his hands, he held it in his mouth. (He claimed years of smoking a pipe helped him with this coordination.) He mentored a teenage boy who wanted to learn to paint. Fearing he would eventually lose his voice (he never did), he made a cassette tape for our grandchildren of the Christmas story from the Bible. The cassette tape carried on a tradition that Doug had kept every Christmas Eve with his own children. It was his last gift to them.

In writing a history of his life for his grandchildren, Doug said, "I have, long ago, come to the conclusion that the only real purpose in my having been born was to be able to pass on to my offspring a value system that would allow them to survive whatever may come their way, and in the process leave this earth a better place for having been here. Somewhere I have read that . . . when you are born you cry and the people around you are happy, so live your life in such a way that when you die you are happy and the people around you cry."

Doug was a gentle, loving, and caring man who loved life and lived it as if he would live forever. As his wife, I and my family are committed to having this book, his legacy to others, circulate as widely as possible. We share an enthusiasm and hope at the prospect of finding a cure for this dreadful disease, as well as the other forty-odd neuro-muscular diseases that afflict so many around the world.

I am deeply grateful to our four daughters and sons-in-law: Laura and Eric, Becky and Mike, Pam and Tom, Kim and Ken, who encouraged me to bring this book to publication. My thanks, also, to Carolyn Nilson, my friend and advisor, my agent Bert Holtje, and to Dr. Nason Hamlin, Dr. Kevin Felice, Elissa Edson, Elanah Sherman, Robert Martin, and Michael Baxa.

In closing, I would like to offer a new motto that I think about each day and that I carry along with the other two:

All is well.
I'm ready for whatever comes today.
My yesterdays have prepared me.

Beverly A. Bucy
Colebrook, Connecticut
June 1996

Preface

Life is terribly deficient in form. Its catastrophes happen in the wrong way and to the wrong people.

—Oscar Wilde

Life is not always what one wants it to be, but to make the best of it as it is, is the only way of being happy.

—Jennie Jerome Churchill

The above two quotes became meaningful to me in October 1992. After several months of complaining about a weak knee joint and assorted other joint-related problems such as weak thumbs, I visited a neurologist at the recommendation of my family physician. After several office visits and an EMG examination at the local hospital, the neurologist came into the examining room and in a rather matter-of-fact manner told me that I had Amyotrophic Lateral Sclerosis (ALS). With a puzzled look I asked him what that meant. To which he replied, "That's Lou Gehrig's disease." That answer didn't give me any more information than his first comment. I told him that I didn't know what that meant either.

He explained to me that Amyotrophic Lateral Sclerosis was a neuro-muscular disease that affected the motor neurons and caused weakness and deterioration of the voluntary muscle groups. I asked him what caused this disease, and he replied, "We don't know." I then asked him, "How is it cured?" His response was, "There is no cure." My next question was, "What is the prognosis?" At that point I was given a "death sentence" of two to five years.

It was at this moment that the quote from Oscar Wilde came rushing into my life. Why me? Why now? I was just 60 years old and felt that my productive energies were at their peak. I drove home that day thinking, if this is all true, why not just drive onto the highway and run my car into the first bridge abutment and be done with it all?

When I arrived home, my wife was out doing errands, and I sat and tried to decided how I was going to tell her the results of the examination without being as cruel as the neurologist had been in his matter-of-fact diagnosis. When she did arrive home, we discussed the situation the best we could. After a long and tearful night, I contacted my family physician who had referred me to the neurologist. We met with him and demanded a second opinion from the most qualified doctor we could find on the East Coast.

That was two years ago, and well, I have made it past the minimum time given to me in October 1992. As will be discussed in greater detail in the following sections, my goal at this time is to leave behind a book to help individuals like myself, who through a wide variety of circumstances find themselves physically disabled and needing help in coping with life in general.

The second quote above is how I have come to look at life now. It is true, that life for me and those around me (my wife, my children, my grandchildren, and my friends) has changed and is continuing to change for us daily. I decided early on that I would make the best of it, even if I only had a year or two left. I have always been a relatively happy man, and life has been good for me. At this point in my life I feel that it doesn't make any sense to make life any more difficult by being unhappy during the time that I have left or making my family and friends any more unhappy than they already are.

Shortly after I was diagnosed with ALS, a long-time friend of mine, a minister, sent me a booklet that sums up my outlook on life. Briefly, it expanded on the story from the New Testament of the Bible where a woman who had a chronic disease sought out Jesus for help. She was unable to get through the crowds of people around him but as Christ passed by, she was only able to touch the hem of his garment. He felt her touch and understood her need, and speaking to her he said, "Your faith has made you whole." My religious faith in God and a hereafter has given me mental strength and mental healing. I have said to many people, "While my faith may not have made me physically whole, it has made me mentally whole." The emotional upheaval caused by this disease has given me a new outlook on life. I intend to live the remainder of my life as if I am going to live forever. If I don't make it that far at least I can live as long as I have, as happily as I can.

One day a few months ago, while I was in a rather "down" mood, I was talking with one of my daughters on the telephone. In response to my remarks that I was feeling rather low, and didn't like what was happening to me, my daughter said, "Well Dad, you could have had a heart attack and died in October 1992, but you are still here with us, and you can still use your mind as well as before. Why don't you think of a way to make it productive as well?"

This set me to thinking about my situation. While the progression of the ALS disease will eventually eliminate my ability to move, leaving me as a quadriplegic, and will ultimately affect my ability to breathe, which will result in death, it will never affect my senses, thoughts, and memory. I suddenly realized that what I was experiencing in progressively varying degrees is similar to that which other people have experienced as a final condition, such as a stroke victim, or someone who has had a spinal injury. While I started out with simple and minor inconveniences and disabilities, the progression of my disease is giving me a full range of disabilities to the point where I am at present, unable to walk, use my hands and arms effectively, and unable to wash or dress myself, and yet I know that I am not close to the final chapter in this episode.

Along the way I have been able to cope with each new phase of the disability by planning ahead and investigating what I will need in order to cope in the future. The idea for this book came to me as I spent many hours on the telephone trying to get my life in order. Making perhaps several hundred telephone calls to various agencies, government bureaus, insurance companies, health aid vendors, doctors, occupational therapists etc., I believe that I have accumulated a wealth of resource data that has been beneficial to me and will hopefully be of assistance to others who encounter similar disabling circumstances. Whether this disability is caused by a disease such as ALS or MS, or initiated by a disabling injury or stroke, the result is very much the same.

This "Help Yourself Guide" makes no pretense of being all inclusive. What I have prepared is primarily based on the first-hand experiences. This book is divided into four major parts. The parts are arranged by types of assistance an individual may require in order to best manage the problems that develop when disability becomes evident. In my particular situation, the problems that I have learned to cope with are those of weakness and loss of function in my hands, feet, arms, legs, and other voluntary muscle groups of the body.

Part I   Deals with help provided by "caregivers."

Part II   Deals with devices and mechanical assistive equipment for managing disability caused by muscular weakness or damage to the central nervous system.

Part III   Deals with help provided by institutions, associations, and other organizations dedicated to assisting the emotional needs of the disabled person and their family.

Part IV   Deals with financial assistance.

I have also researched topics and concerns that were of little relevance to my personal situation. I have tried to prepare a full range of resource contacts with telephone numbers and addresses. Throughout the text I have included the addresses and telephone numbers of various agencies, associations, organizations, and, in some cases, vendors that have been helpful.

The primary point that I would like to impress upon you at this time, is that you and only you can take charge of your life. You must be your own advocate! You can receive help from professional advocates in almost every area of need; however, you must be in the driver's seat. Not only will this give you quicker and more efficient results, it will give you a sense of continued independence. This is perhaps the hardest lesson that I had to learn. My progressively debilitating disease is robbing me of my independence. To give up my independence and to learn patience have for me been the most difficult barriers to overcome.

Professor Morris Schwartz at Brandeis University, having also been diagnosed with Lou Gehrig's disease, has written a book titled *Reflections on Maintaining One's Composure While Living with a Fatal Illness*. In this book he says, "Begin by asserting a willful determination to be composed." By being composed, Professor Schwartz does not mean keeping a stiff upper lip or hiding your feelings, or trying to be self-contained. "Composure," Dr. Schwartz says, "consists of one or more of the following qualities: high spirits, inner peacefulness, courage, dignity, open-heartedness, humor, nobility, life-affirming patience, involvement, self-respect, and self-esteem."

In this book I have attempted to show how disabled individuals can achieve composure by taking charge of their lives and solving the problems that arise while trying to cope with a drastically altered situations.

The sections devoted to caregivers have, for the most part, been firsthand experiences. I cannot even begin to fully explain to my devoted wife how she has eased the emotional catastrophe that struck our household two years ago. Without her love and comfort this experience would be one of terror and unbearable misery. The support of my family during this time has, likewise, been great. Our friends and associates in the Church and community have given both myself and my wife support and strength.

Douglas R. Bucy
Colebrook, Connecticut
June 1995

Acknowledgments

I wish to acknowledge and thank all of my family, friends, and neighbors who have encouraged and assisted me in the completion of this book. Without the help of people like Shirley Fredlund, of the Voice for Joannie program, who provided me with the voice-activated computer system, I would have had a monumental job of putting my thoughts on paper; and our friend Carolyn Nilson, who from the outset has pointed me in the right directions and has encouraged me to complete this book.

My daughter Rebecca Nolan worked with me, preparing the illustrations that I feel add much to the understanding of the material presentation. My daughter Pam Ragonese at the very outset has prodded me forward and has been helpful in doing some detailed research work. My other two daughters, Laura Hesterberg and Kim Gutkowski, have both been supportive and have provided good "sounding board" feedback on the direction that the book has taken. Further, I wish to thank Betsey Audette and Tom Voorhees for their assistance in preparing some of the resource material.

Finally, I want to take special note of my wife Bev, caregiver, rewriter, material sorter, critic, devil's advocate, prodder, and all-around assistant, for her support, without which I could not have achieved the goal we set for ourselves.

Part • I
Caregivers

C h a p t e r • 1

The Primary Caregiver

"IN SICKNESS AND IN HEALTH . . . UNTIL DEATH DO US PART"

When we committed to this marriage vow 40 years ago, my wife and I never gave any real thought to what it might mean to us in the future. Yet here we are today facing a fatal disease that worsens each day. Dr. John Rolland from the Center for Family Health at the University of Chicago writes in the *Journal of Marital and Family Therapy* that most couples who are about to become married usually give little thought to what a life together with an illness or a disability would be like. According to Dr. Rolland, an illness or a disability can often damage marriages, even the strongest and sturdiest ones. When an illness or a disability occurs, couples are forced to reexamine all aspects of their relationship and restructure their lives without really knowing what to expect. Dr. Rolland further writes that the healthy partner often suffers from "survivor's guilt," the feeling that he/she doesn't deserve any more than his/her sick or disabled partner.

Former First Lady Rosalynn Carter states in her most recent book, *Helping Yourself Help Others*,[1] that 80 percent of informal caregivers are women. Of this group of women, an overwhelming majority are the patient's spouse. My wife, my primary caregiver, has like myself had to adjust different conditions almost on a daily basis. Like other caregivers, she faces a daily dose of little privacy, physical exhaustion, isolation, loneliness, and guilt. However, she has learned to cope with these conditions by reserving some private time for herself and by maintaining outside interests. The disease that I have, ALS (or Lou Gehrig's disease), is a progressive disease which causes motor control muscles to weaken. The various stages of deterioration constantly pose new challenges for my caregiver and more obstacles for me in my ongoing attempt to live an independent life. Part II describes in detail how my wife and I coped with each hurdle that surfaced. The following sections briefly address some of the difficulties that we encountered and ways we dealt with them. Keep in mind as you read that each individual must a problem-solving plan that will work for his or her particular situation.

"IT MUST HAVE GONE DOWN HARD"

During one Sunday morning service while speaking on the subject of pride, our minister used the following anecdote to make her point:

> The headlight of her car burned out and required a replacement. Since she was very handy and somewhat mechanically inclined, she decided to change the light herself rather than go to a service garage. Removing the lamp proved to be a simple task. The new light was installed and only needed the locknut to be tightened. However, after numerous attempts to fasten the locknut, resulting in bloody knuckles and a split fingernail, she decided to give up and call for help. A friend of hers, living not too far away, had volunteered numerous times in the past to help her with projects she could not do. She called him and in less time than it took him to drive to her home, he had the locknut tightened. In thanking him she said, "I had to swallow my pride before I called you." His reply was, "It must have gone down hard."

This anecdote points out that we must all be willing to swallow our pride, no matter how hard it goes down, and ask for help from those around us who are more than willing to assist us if we only ask.

In her book *Keys to Survival for Caregivers*,[2] Mary Kouri remarks, "No matter what your relationship was like in the past, your illness or disability is likely to upset the division of skills and responsibilities between you and your spouse." She further lists some of the areas that become chaotic for many couples:

finances

housekeeping

repairs

yard work

shopping

automobile maintenance

In each of these areas, I had to learn how to swallow my pride and ask for assistance from others. For example, during my entire married life I was responsible for handling my family's finances. During the early stages of my disability, I continued to take on this responsibility. As time went on, however, it became more difficult for me to physically handle invoices, sort bills, and write checks. Soon it became evident that I needed to shift our family's financial responsibilities to my wife.

In the past, I also handled household repair and yard work projects myself. Unfortunately, as I became less able to handle tools and use the stairs to my basement workshop, the repair tasks either went untended or were handled by hired help. In time, my four sons-in-law began to handle the repair jobs around the house. Without my family's support in this area as well, these projects would have been postponed, become very costly to resolve, and become sources of depression and personal frustration.

As will be discussed later in more detail, it is important to maintain open lines of communication with your family and friends. In my situation, my wife and I maintained close family contact throughout the progression of my disease. Our family and friends have helped us meet emotional and physical needs, and have lightened the load that my wife has had to assume. The support from our family and friends, however, was not initiated by them. Instead, we received the help we needed by relinquishing our pride, opening our lives to them, and clearly informing them of what we needed.

Lastly, some tasks are best handled by friends or relatives who often ask "How can I help?" If you have friends or relatives that offer vague help, begin keeping a list of things that need to be done which you and your caregiver don't have the time, energy, or ability to handle yourselves. Then, when people genuinely offer their services, let them select an item or two from your list. This provides a focus for everyone involved.

For more information on obtaining support, contact the Well Spouse Foundation whose motto is "When one is sick . . . two need help." This helpful organization can be reached at:

Well Spouse Foundation
YWCA
610 Lexington Avenue
Room 814
New York, NY 10022
(212) 644-1241
(800) 838-0879 (toll-free 24-hour answering machine)

"WALK IN MY SHOES FOR A MILE OR SO"

Throughout the course of my illness, there have certainly been times when I have not seen eye to eye with my caregiver. This lack of consensus has occurred on many issues. Unfortunately, it has always been difficult for my wife and me to talk about problems that trouble us, and the "terminal" prognosis of my disease has not helped the situation. However, my wife's ability to "read" me and understand my needs and frustrations has compensated for our lack of verbal communication. There are several emotions that I continue to experience as my disability worsens. I am sure that other people with disabilities also experience these emotions as well:

Fear The fear of losing control over my physical functions;

The fear of losing control over my personal life;

And, mostly, the fear of the unknown. I'm not afraid of dying, but I am afraid of not knowing exactly how I will die.

Fear is sometimes masked by other emotions such as anger or impatience. It is up to the caregiver to draw out the disabled person's buried feelings.

Sadness I enjoy life very much and am sad about the prospect of it being cut short. I have been fortunate enough to see my immediate family grow to adulthood with families of their own, but now I'm selfish in wanting to see my grandchildren also grow up. I suppose that no matter how old a person becomes, there is always something in the future he/she wants to witness. Therefore, knowing that I won't be alive to see many things happen makes me sad.

Anger I, at times, become angry and frustrated with the difficulties and inconveniences caused by my disability.

Being totally dependent on another person for every day needs generates emotions and feelings that are not usually felt and are difficult to explain. It is therefore easy for the disabled person to begin demanding more from his or her caregiver and to begin finding fault with the caregiver's efforts. My five-year-old grandson expressed it best one day when he said to his mother, "I know that sometimes when you're angry with me or Sister or when you get mad at Daddy, you are really feeling sad because of your daddy."

OUTSIDE INTERESTS

As previously mentioned, it is important that caregivers participate in activities outside of the home. This allows them time to take their minds off their responsibilities and focus on events completely separate and different. Caregivers must maintain a balance between their caregiving responsibilities and the need to sustain their own individualities. Prior to my illness, my wife was involved in several activities at our church. She was also involved in our town's historical society and was the deputy registrar for the voting commission. As my condition worsened, we talked at length about her ability to stay involved in these outside functions. We decided that as long as I am able to remain relatively self-sufficient, she should continue to take part in these activities. As a result, my wife has something to look forward to outside of our home and activities to plan for each week.

TAKING TIME OUT

A health care professional told me that one of the greatest problems in coping with a disability is its potential effect on the caregiver. Since caregivers may end up feeling overwhelmed, it is important to make arrangements to receive extra help early. When I discussed this with my wife, she said in a rather off-handed manner, "Oh, I don't think that I will need any help." Nevertheless the situation bothered me, and I was determined to arrange for temporary relief or respite for her before the daily stress of caregiving overwhelmed her.

Today, with my daughters' help, my wife has at least one day each week when she is relieved of her caregiving responsibilities. One of my daughters comes on a weekly basis and spends five to six hours with me, while another visits every other week for an afternoon and evening. A third daughter who works full time in a neighboring town comes for an hour or so each Friday. In addition to my daughters, I have several friends who help out. Between my daughters and friends, my wife is able to take a respite one or two days each week. Currently, we are trying to make arrangements that will allow her to take an overnight or weekend visit away at least once a month.

Besides family and friends, there are services that can offer aid to your caregiver. Some services you may want to consider are:

Regular or occasional adult day care centers. For example, some nursing home facilities may provide day care as a supplement to their regular long-term health care services.

Home health care or hospice professionals. Contact your local Visiting Nurse Association for more information.

Temporary nursing homes or senior citizen's residences. These are possible longer term solutions for more than one or two nights.

These services, though, are not cheap. For example, a one day's stay at a hospice can cost as much as $50 in my community. However, Medicare and some private insurance may cover at least a portion of the costs. In addition, the Veterans Administration (VA) provides respite care in VA hospitals for eligible veterans, and some community and local agencies offer respite programs and grants. Again, contact your local Visiting Nurse Association for more information.

The key to remember here is to *plan to find help before you need help*. Taking care of a person on a full-time basis is a very demanding responsibility that gets harder and tougher to handle down the road.

TAKING CARE OF THE CAREGIVER

Taking care of yourself as a caregiver may seem at first like a selfish idea. It may be difficult for you to see how taking care of yourself will benefit your charge. At one time or another, you've probably witnessed an overworked teacher or nurse grow impatient. This impatience is what can happen to quality care when a person becomes overworked and exhausted. A short pamphlet titled "Caring for Yourself When You're Caring for Someone Ill"[3] lists a number of self-care tips:

Pace yourself	Although you may be strong and independent, you are not superhuman. You must acknowledge your limitations and learn to ask for help. Make a list of things that need to be done and ask your family and friends for their assistance while leaving them the option to say no.
Acknowledge your strengths	Give yourself credit every day for the work that you perform. Your patient may be too overwhelmed by his/her illness to fully express his/her appreciation for all that you are doing.
Talk it over	As a caregiver, you also need someone to care for you. Find someone with whom you can safely discuss your feelings and needs, such as a friend, counselor, or pastor.

Nurture your body   Caregivers tend to ignore their own physical needs. Eating well and exercising are often the last things that they think about at the end of an exhausting day. However, keeping fit and healthy is not only beneficial for the patient, but it will also help you maintain a positive outlook on life.

Caring for someone can be quite challenging but yet rewarding. My relationship with my wife has become more meaningful as we continue to face my illness together. Her help has made the concept of death less fearsome for me. Caregivers, though, can only commit to caring for others if they take care of themselves too.

Support Groups

My doctor had suggested numerous times that my wife attend support group meetings with me. My wife and I, however, felt that we had everything under control and did not need "outside" help. After finally attending one meeting, we discovered a group of people who really understood each other. We learned that our emotions were not unique and that these people also sometimes felt angry, frustrated, impatient, and fearful. My wife especially benefited from these support groups. She met other spouses who at times were just as emotionally drained as she. For a listing of support groups in your area, refer to the listing of volunteer health agencies in Part III.

Handling Stress

Stress is a term used to describe the body's and mind's reactions to everyday tensions and pressures. Everyone at one time or another has probably experienced a faster heartbeat, higher blood pressure, shortness of breath, and muscle stiffness. These physical changes are indications that the body is preparing for activities that require added strength and energy. Stress can be compared to a violin string: If it is too loose, it won't produce music; however, if the string is too tight, it will break. Some degree of stress is necessary to function properly, however, too much stress build-up can harm your body. *Coping With Stress*, distributed by the National Multiple Sclerosis Society,[4] lists the following as symptoms of too much stress:

    Tiredness/exhaustion
    Muscle tension
    Anxiety
    Ingestion
    Nervousness/trembling

Sleeplessness

Cold, sweaty hands

Reduced or increased appetite

Grinding teeth/clenching jaws

General body complaints such as weakness, dizziness, headache, stomachache, or back pain

Since stress is a part of everyday living, especially for caregivers who usually experience an exorbitant amount of stress, it is important to recognize the signs of stress early and learn to cope effectively. Handling stress is not eliminating stress, but it is knowing how to manage it. One way to manage stress is by learning to relax. Relaxing is more than just sitting back and remaining silent. Instead, relaxing should be an active process. One way to relax is to exercise since the increase in oxygen intake tends to alleviate tense muscles. Walking is recognized as one of the best forms of exercise for all ages. It can be practiced anywhere, no special equipment is needed, and it can be done alone or with a group. Caregivers may make a formal exercise out of walking by setting a specific course to walk or they can make it as informal as parking their car at the furthest part of a shopping center lot and walking the additional distance. Exercise is also recognized as a cure for sleeplessness, ingestion, muscle tension, and anxiety—all symptoms of stress.

Another way a caregiver may relax is to have an in-house diversion. My wife, for example, uses knitting, cross-stitch needlework, computer solitaire, and occasional crossword puzzles as activities in our home to help her cope with stress. I try to avoid interrupting her as she participates in these diversions since they are a vital part of her physical and mental well-being.

Dealing with Anger and Guilt

I'm not sure which of these two emotions is experienced first, but I do know that all caregivers experience them. Flashes of anger can come without any warning and, in many cases, with justification. My oftentimes irritating habits and poorly timed requests (viewed sometimes as demands), coupled with uncompleted tasks and other demands, often cause my caregiver to lash out in anger. Constructive management of anger can help caregivers and patients cope with the underlying problem, which is the illness or disability, and not the patients themselves. One way to manage anger is to schedule frequent breaks. This recess will allow caregivers to gather their thoughts, refocus, and recharge.

Like anger, guilt is a natural emotion felt by the caregiver. The caregiver can easily become overwhelmed with too many obligations, which often result in uncompleted tasks. Like many caregivers, my wife was quite energetic when she first began taking care of me. Often, caregivers surprise themselves with their own skills and stamina. Their survival instinct kicks in, and despite a lack of rest, the caregiver feels alert and responsive. While our survival instinct is designed to get us through a short-term crisis, it does not work on a long-term basis. As things are left undone, caregivers begin to feel guilty and wonder if what they are doing is enough. Unless this guilt is resolved, the caregiver will begin to feel burned out. Caregivers must learn to let go of their fantasies of "perfection" and not hold themselves accountable for unrealistic goals or standards. One of the best ways to keep caregiving free from guilt is to join a support group where other caregivers will help keep things in better perspective.

Professional
Caregivers

MEDICAL SPECIALISTS

Although the disabled person's family physician usually serves as his or her first point of contact, the patient is usually referred to specialists. There are more than twenty-two specialties recognized by the American Medical Association. Although many types of medical specialists may become involved in the treatment and rehabilitation of a disabled individual, there are six specialties which play key roles.

Physical Medicine and Rehabilitation

Specialists in this area combine physical medicine and rehabilitation with a basic training in medicine, physiology, pathology, biochemistry, pharmacology, and behavioral and social sciences. The rehabilitation specialist shares with other physicians the general skills and knowledge required of all medical practitioners. This knowledge, combined with therapeutic aids such as drugs, exercise, and medical or motorized devices, helps patients acquire the best possible medical and physical conditions. This specialist may assume complete medical responsibility for general as well as special care or may act only as a consultant.

Psychiatrists

Psychiatrists are physicians who specialize in the diagnosis, treatment, and prevention of mental and emotional disorders. In a rehabilitation center, a psychiatrist may study the effects of a physical disability on a patient's personality. In addition, psychologists and case managers often consult psychiatrists regarding a patient's particular treatment program.

Neurologists

A neurologist, or nerve specialist, diagnoses and treats organic diseases and disorders of the nervous system such as epilepsy, multiple sclerosis, Amyotrophic Lateral Sclerosis, Charcot-Marie-Tooth disease, Guillain-Barré syndrome, polio, spinal cord injuries, strokes, and Parkinson's disease.

Orthopedists

An orthopedist, or orthopedic surgeon, treats diseases and deformities of the spine, bones, joints, muscles, or other parts of the skeletal system through the use of medical, surgical, and physical therapy procedures. The disorders may be congenital or acquired from an illness or injury, and can include such disabling conditions as spinal curvature, clubfoot, hip dysplasia, foot drop, amputations, Muscular Dystrophy, osteoporosis, and arthritis.

Ophthalmologists

An ophthalmologist, or eye physician, diagnoses and treats diseases of and injuries to the eyes, many of which lead to a chronic reduction in sight or a complete loss of sight requiring special rehabilitative measures. Disorders of the eyes include cataracts, glaucoma, detached retina, ophthalmia neonatorum, and retinitis pigmentosa. An eye specialist determines the nature and extent of the disorder, prescribes and administers appropriate medication, performs surgery such as corneal transplantation, and executes a variety of tests to determine the loss of vision. Ophthalmologists also direct medical and rehabilitative procedures designed to improve sight or fully utilize the remaining sight. This treatment may include writing prescriptions for corrective glasses or contact lenses and instructing patients in care of and exercises for the eye.

Radiologists

Radiologists specialize in the use of X-rays and radioactive substances in diagnosis and therapy. They take X-ray pictures, or radiographs, which then are used to reveal and evaluate such conditions as skull fractures, bone injuries, malignant or nonmalignant tumors, or cardiac enlargement.

RELATED SPECIALISTS

Social Workers

A social worker is an integral and essential member of any rehabilitation team. This person is a highly skilled specialist who helps individuals and families deal with personal problems that arise when they are faced with illness or disability. These problems may be work related, or involve a family's finances, living arrangements, social life, marriage, or child care. Since these problems are usually complex, a special knowledge and expertise are necessary to handle them.

Since a social worker plays a fundamental role in the life of a disabled person and his/her family, choose a social worker with the same care you would use when choosing a physician. First of all, make sure to select a *professional* social worker. This may be tricky since the title "social worker" is not a "protected" title. In other professions, for example, only persons with a specific degree can call themselves "physicians" or "nurses." However, people who have no formal training can call themselves "social workers." It is critically important that a social worker possess a Bachelor's degree in Social Work (B.S.W.) or a Master's degree in Social Work (M.S.W.) If the social worker does not have either of these two degrees, or worse, no degree at all, you should carefully question that person's ability to provide the care and assistance required. In addition, some states require that social workers be certified or licensed. A certified social worker usually has an M.S.W. degree.

When meeting a social worker for the first time, find out the extent of training completed and related experience as well as the following:

- What community services are available, and does the social worker know how to help you obtain their assistance?
- Is the social worker familiar with your insurance coverage and whether it is adequate for meeting the expenses of managing your disability. If it is not sufficient, does the social worker know what other financial arrangements you can make to meet your expenses?
- Is the social worker prepared to give direct care? Direct care is "hands on" treatment and participation in the patient's case. In other words, is this professional a "clinical" social worker? While most persons with an M.S.W. perform clinical social work directly with patients, some are "administrative" social workers. The disabled patient needs the services of a "hands on" clinical social worker rather than an administrator.

- Does the social worker know how you can secure home health care? Many chronic diseases are generally managed in the home and patients often need help from aides and nurses. The social worker must be able to put you in touch with these people if you need them.

- You also need to find out early on what the social worker cannot do. The social worker works within the established "system" and sometimes just can't acquire all the help a patient may need. Don't assume that the social worker can solve all your problems. It is important to re-emphasize here that **you are ultimately responsible for meeting your needs.** The social worker can usually assist only in finding the right help for you at the right time. It is also important to stress that you must be persistent in making your needs known. If a need is refused or ignored, try again. **Don't take no for an answer!**

Physical Therapists

Physical therapists play an essential role in the rehabilitation of the physically disabled. They are responsible for administering treatments designed to alleviate a patient's pain, correct or minimize deformities, show a patient how to use assistive and supportive devices, and increase a patient's strength and mobility.

The following is a sampling of specific activities as outlined in the Disability and Rehabilitation Handbook[5] for which the physical therapist has primary responsibility: planning and supervision of individualized treatment programs; application of testing and evaluation procedures; recording and reporting results of these procedures; evaluating orthotic and prosthetic devices; supervising or carrying out a predetermined exercise program; development of ambulatory and elevation skills; training in the use of braces, crutches, prostheses, and other assistive and supportive devices; application of specialized treatment procedures, such as hot and cold packs, paraffin, moist air, infrared, diathermy, ultrasound, ultraviolet, massage, traction, vascular apparatus, and electrodiagnosis and treatment; application of specified hydrotherapy treatment, such as whirlpool, Hubbard tank, contrast baths, and therapeutic pools.

The practice of physical therapy is regulated in every state. All physical therapists require a license or registration on the basis of a state examination. The American Physical Therapy Association establishes the accreditation standards for physical therapy educational programs. To contact them for more information, write to:

The American Physical Therapy Association
1156 Fifteenth Street N.W.
Washington, DC 20005

Occupational Therapists

Occupational therapists assist patients in adapting to their environment and in handling daily living activities with the maximum amount of independence. Occupational therapy services may be provided in the home, hospital, rehabilitation center, outpatient clinic, special school settings, nursing home, or work environment.

Respiratory Therapists

Respiratory therapy, also known as inhalation therapy, is an allied health occupation based on the administration of oxygen and other gases and mists for medical purposes. The responsibilities of the respiratory therapist include not only the actual administration of inhalants in the most suitable manner, but also include explaining the treatment to the patient and caregiver, instructing in the use of equipment, products, and procedures, as well as regulating gas flow during treatments. The therapist is also required to teach patients and caregivers how to keep the equipment clean, sterile, and in good working condition.

Orthotists and Prosthetists

These two occupations are grouped together because they require the same training and skills, and in many cases hold the same responsibilities. A prosthetist makes and fits artificial limbs for amputees, while the orthotist makes and fits orthopedic braces to support or correct body parts weakened or distorted by disease or injury. Both work directly under a physician's supervision. Once a device is made and fitted, a physical or occupational therapist then helps the patient learn how to use it.

Homemakers/Home Health Aides

A homemaker/home health aide is a paraprofessional who is recruited, trained, and professionally supervised by an employing community agency such as a Visiting Nurse Association, a hospital with a home care unit, or a public health or social service department. They assist patients with bathing, performing prescribed exercises, and using prosthetic equipment.

Homemaker/home health aide services began early in this century as a way to help families with young children during a mother's illness or convalescence. Over the years the service grew to encompass the needs of the physically and mentally ill, the elderly, and disabled persons of all ages.

Visiting Nurses and Home Care Services

Next to the primary caregiver, the Visiting Nurse Association is perhaps the most valuable outside agency in terms of offering assistance to patients. The Visiting Nurse and Home Care Services organizations usually consist of the following professionals:

Public Health Nurses

Dietitians

Physical Therapists

Homemakers/Home Health Aides

Medical Social Workers

Occupational Therapists

Speech Therapists

These professionals form a team approach to home medical care. The goal of the Visiting Nurse Association is to help the patient regain his or her maximum health potential as quickly as possible while providing invaluable support to the patient's family during the illness and rehabilitation. These two organizations help to:

- Teach the patient's family how to provide care between visits.
- Instruct the patient and caregiver to properly use and care for medical equipment.
- Monitor the patient's condition and maintain contact with the responsible physician.
- Coordinate health and social services needed to assure complete care.
- Give special treatments as prescribed by the physician including services by a registered nurse, a licensed practical nurse, or a licensed vocational nurse under the supervision of an RN.
- Assist with physical rehabilitation, which may involve treatment to relieve pain, restore movement, and regain strength.
- Offer counseling on good nutrition and advice on special diets and meal planning.

Costs for these services are usually covered by Medicare, Medicaid, Blue Cross, or other insurance policies. For those unable to pay, services are provided for a partial fee or at no charge as long as funds are available. Note, for home health care services to be covered by Medicare, you must need at least one of the following three services:

1. Part-time skilled nursing care

2. Physical therapy

3. Speech therapy

If any of these three types of therapy are required, Medicare may also cover occupational therapy and medical social services.

PART I NOTES

1. Rosalynn Carter and Susan K. Golant, *Helping Yourself Help Others* (New York, Times Books).

2. Mary K. Kouri, Ph.D., *Keys to Survival for Caregivers* (New York, Barron's Educational Series, 1992).

3. "Caring for Yourself When You're Caring for Someone Ill," CareNotes (Abbey Press, St. Meinrad, IN, publication No. 50–21272–0).

4. "Coping With Stress," National Multiple Sclerosis Society, Chicago/North Illinois Chapter.

5. Robert M. Goldstein, ed., *Disibility and Rehabilitation Handbook* (McGraw-Hill, 1990).

Part • II

Day-to-Day
Living

Independent Living

As my disease progressed, it became more and more strenuous for me to perform my daily activities satisfactorily. For example, walking became laborious
and dressing myself became a long, backbreaking process since the range of
motion in my arms, hands, and shoulders decreased significantly. In addition,
my fingers lost dexterity, making the use of eating utensils extremely difficult to
control. After discussing these problems with my physical and occupational
therapists, I realized that there are five stages to what we term "dependency."

Independent	Independent individuals are able to continue working and perform self-care tasks and household activities. However, they may experience some difficulty in carrying out these tasks. For instance, these individuals may experience fatigue and weakness in particular muscle groups, such as in the knees and thumbs.
Independent with Assistive Devices	Weakness of the small muscle groups of the hands and the arms make certain self-care, household, and occupa-tional tasks more difficult for individuals in this stage. This weakness, combined with increased fatigue, may require individuals to use assistive devices such as a cane for walking.
Mini Assistance	As weakness increases in the hands, shoulders, or feet as well as in other muscles, activities such as cutting meat, opening doors, and holding articles become quite arduous for individuals. Combing one's hair, climbing stairs, and rising from a chair all become very difficult to do alone.
Major Assistance	Individuals in this stage of dependency have such significant weakness in the arms and legs that the use

of both assistive devices and the help of another person is necessary. For example, individuals who use wheelchairs may also need assistance getting into and out of one.

Dependent   Severe weakness of the limbs, neck, and trunk forces individuals in this stage to rely on their caregiver to help them perform all tasks.

Together, my caregivers and I determined that the use of assistive devices designed to help disabled people perform various muscle movements was necessary. The following sections will describe the most commonly used assistive devices. Keep in mind that you and your physical and/or occupational therapist must decide and identify which devices will be most useful and beneficial for you. Also keep in mind that your situation is likely to change fairly often, and this consideration is not to be taken lightly.

There are two types of assistive devices. The first type of device modifies the things we use every day so that they are less difficult to operate and handle. For example, forks and spoons with added padding on their handles make them easier to manipulate and more comfortable. Adding hand straps to brushes and combs allows a person with a weak grasp to continue performing normal grooming activities. In addition, specially designed items such as cups and plates, doorknobs and other similar tools often have easy-to-use substitutes or modifications.

The second type of device is actually added to an individual's body to support joints and help maintain positions that the muscles can no longer maintain by themselves. These personal devices help people preserve the ability to complete the tasks of active daily living.

DAILY LIVING AIDS

Eating Aids

Eating has always been one of my favorite activities. During the early stages of my disease, there was little indication that I would have any trouble eating normally. However, as my disease progressed, my hands and arms weakened considerably making utensils more difficult to use. Consequently, eating became less an enjoyable activity and more a strenuous task. The following pages feature some devices I used to help make the process of eating easier and more manageable.

Figure 1 features the scoop dish that contains a rolled side which serves as a wall for sliding food onto utensils. The dish also has a deep inner lip which helps prevent spills.

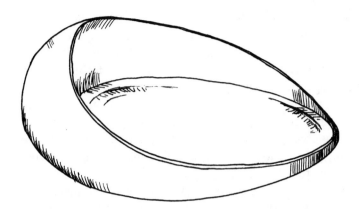

Figure 1   Scoop Dish

Plate guards, shown in figure 2, snap onto any plate rim. Plate guards prevent spills by keeping food on the plate.

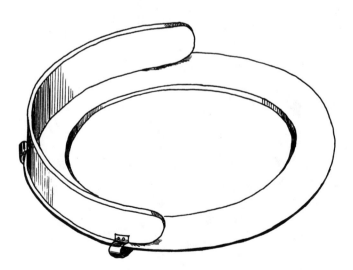

Figure 2   Plate Guards

For those who have trouble keeping their plates in a stationary position, high-quality melamine bowls with suction bases are available. By turning a lever on the lock-tight suction base the bowl is held securely in place on any smooth surface. This is a valuable device for anyone with limited or decreased motor coordination.

In addition to suction-base dishes, nonslip pads and placemats are ideal additions to any table setting. They come in a number of precut sizes and shapes and some have self-adhesive backing which adheres to most surfaces.

Slow eaters may find a plastic hotplate useful. This insulated dish contains a bottom compartment that holds hot or cold liquid that keeps food at serving temperature throughout the meal. And for those who find consuming sandwiches too demanding, metal tongs and plastic holders are available. These devices, however, require some degree of arm strength to be used effectively. Unfortunately, as my hands deteriorated so did my arms, making sandwiches still quite difficult for me to eat.

Utensils, for me, are especially hard to control and manage. My ability to hold a standard knife or fork is limited, and instead I have found utensils with enlarged handles (such as those shown in figure 3) much easier to use. These utensils may be purchased with steel cylinders or foam-rubber handles.

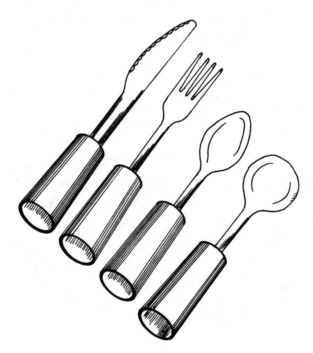

Figure 3 Utensils

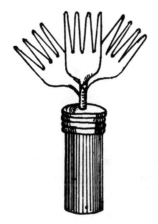

Figure 4   Special Utensil—Fork

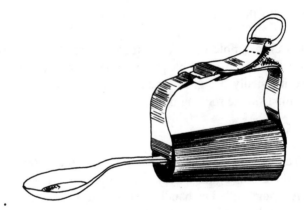

Figure 5   Special Utensil—Spoon with strap

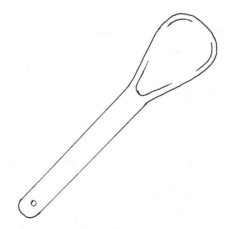

Figure 6   Special Utensil—Spoon

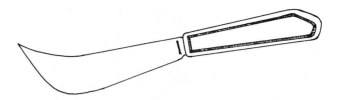

Figure 7 Rocker Knife

Some utensils also come with angled or swiveling handles (figure 4) which can bend up to 90 degrees either to the left or right. These unique utensils with flexible ribbed handles conform to the user's grip and assist persons with a limited range of motion in their hands. In addition, a cuff (shown in figure 5) may be attached to a spoon or fork. This utensil holder is ideal for those with minimal hand strength. The cuff's hook, loop, and D-ring allow users to both slip on and take off the cuff as well as adjust the size easily. Figure 6 shows a spoon.

Figure 6 is an example of a "care spoon," one that is designed with a narrow, shallow bowl. These durable plastic spoons provide protection for teeth and gums. The unusually designed "rocker knife," shown in figure 7, makes cutting easy with a simple rocking motion.

Drinking Aids

For those who are able to maintain some degree of hand dexterity and strength, ordinary cups and drinking glasses may be modified for easier use. For example, figure 8 features mugs with dual handles. These mugs provide two-angled hand grips which enable the user to hold the cup at a proper drinking angle even with diminished grip and muscle control. Another similar type of mug has a wide, nonskid base and a wide handle for an easy full-handed grip. In addition, vacuum-feeding cups are available for those who need assistance in sipping and drinking. These cups prevent dribbling and spilling by enabling the user to control the flow of liquid intake with a soft rubber button.

Personal Hygiene Aids

There are many personal hygiene assistive devices available that include everything from specially designed toenail clippers to $24^{1}/_{2}$-inch-long foot brushes. One instrument I find especially helpful as my hand dexterity continues to diminish is the electric toothbrush. A dental floss holder is also a perfect substitute for hand/finger-held dental floss. Similarly, a toothbrush holder that contains a hand strap is an effective tool for persons with sufficient arm strength. Also available are the automatic toothpaste dispenser and the "toothpaste tube squeeze key," which both make toothpaste more accessible.

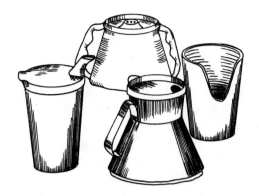

Figure 8   Drinking Glasses

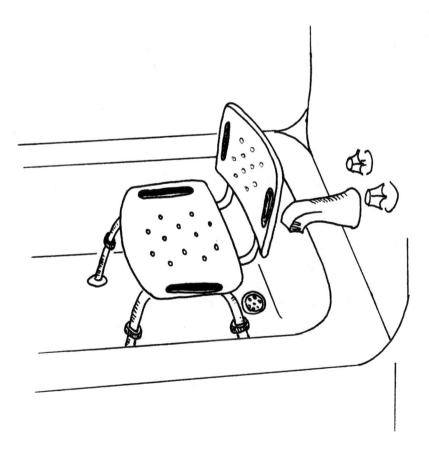

Figure 9   Bath Stool

Daily showers or baths have become a daily "adventure" as my disease progresses. Getting into and out of a shower or tub is a very risky activity even with the help of others since the chance of slipping and falling is a constant danger. The free-standing shower stool or chair is a necessity for any individual with diminished leg strength. The one shown in figure 9 is only one of the many types of bathtub seats and shower chairs available. Personal selection should be based on individual needs and preferences.

Some consideration should be given to height adjustability of bath stools. As the weakness in my legs increases, my shower/tub seat needs to be appropriately adjusted so that I can stand with minimal help. There are a number of assistive devices that provide for various degrees of mobility. Some of these devices are very sophisticated such as the aquatic bathtub lifter which is quite expensive and is not covered by any medical insurance. However, other devices as simple as bathtub rails and tub grab bars (see figure 10) also provide support for users entering and exiting showers/tubs. Usually, these devices have textured finishes for a nonslip grip.

In addition, disabled persons may purchase bathboards or safety benches which both provide extra support for bathers. Lastly, shower and bathtub safety treads or mats, shower extensions, back scrubbers, and soap mitts all make shower or bath use much safer and more enjoyable.

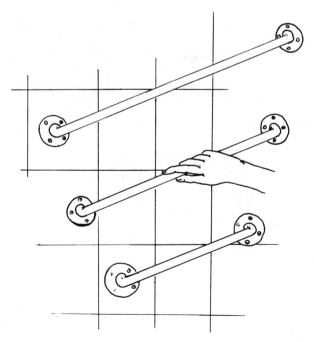

Figure 10   Grab Bars

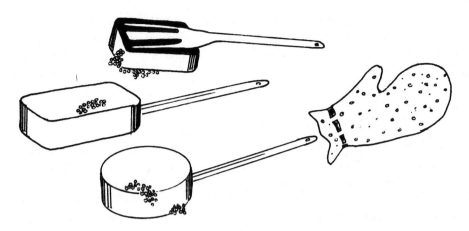

Figure 11   Bath Mitt and Scrubbers

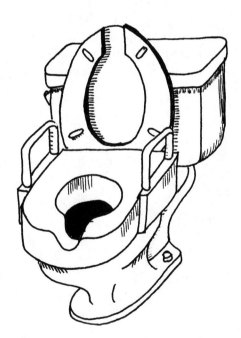

Figure 12   Toilet Seat Extender

Raised toilet seats that fit onto any standard toilet seat enable users with weakened leg muscles to raise and lower themselves with ease. Most models have a molded plastic seat that is 4 to 5 inches in height and some models also have armrests (figure 12). Elevated wall-mounted toilet bowls and manual or hydraulic elevated toilet seats are two permanent devices that are also available and should be considered.

Unfortunately, I was not able to find a permanent device to aid me with the use of a toilet. I have discovered that as my physical condition changes and worsens, what had worked previously no longer meets my needs. It is important that individuals work closely with their occupational therapists in choosing effective equipment.

Dressing Aids

Since I was losing muscle strength in my thumbs and dexterity in my fingers, I had difficulty buttoning shirt buttons. After seeing an occupational therapist regularly, I obtained a button/zipper-hook pull combo (figure 13) which simply slips through a button hole and grasps the button while pulling it back through the hole. The zipper hook grasps the zipper tab, enabling users to pull it up and down. Other simple devices, such as rings or leather thongs that are placed on the zipper, make zipping jackets much easier.

A long-handled shoehorn that ranges from 12 to 30 inches long, as shown in figure 14, lets users put their shoes on without having to bend over. Figure 15 features a stocking pull-on aid that helps individuals slip their sock over a guide and then insert their foot into the sock. By pulling on the attached strap, users are able to draw the sock over their heels and upward onto their calves.

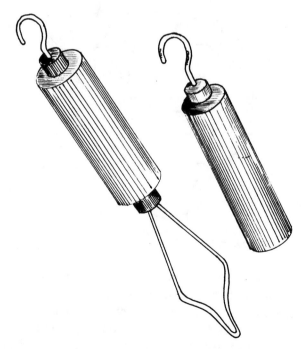

Figure 13   Button/Zipper Hook

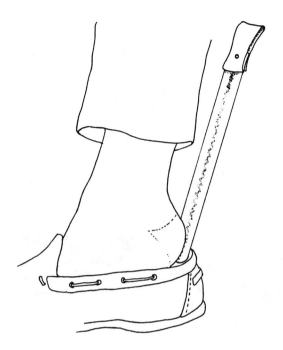

Figure 14 Shoehorns

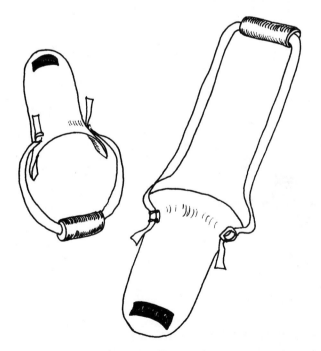

Figure 15 Sock Pull-ons

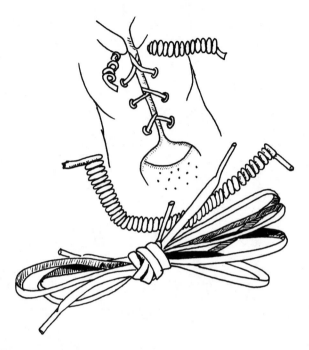

Figure 16   Elastic Shoelaces

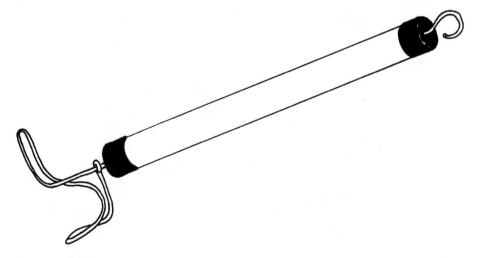

Figure 17   Dressing Stick

Elastic shoelaces, like those shown in figure 16, eliminate any fumbling with shoelaces since they are permanently tied and laced onto the shoe (by someone with good motor skills). These elastic shoelaces stay secure and comfortable since they easily expand and contract. Another handy shoe-tool to obtain is the boot jack, which helps users remove their shoes.

The dressing stick, featured in figure 17, assists those with decreased hip flexion or limited upper extremity movement dress themselves. The stick, made from wood or plastic, contains a metal hook-end and a push/pull end that is over two feet long. This design makes it efficient to use with all types of clothing. Even after not being able to dress myself any longer, I found it to be a valuable tool to have for turning on wall-mounted light switches or for hooking items to retrieve.

Grooming Aids

Grooming was an important part of my daily preparation while I was still able to work outside of my home. When my wrists and arms became too weak to use a standard razor, I obtained an electric one. However, I soon became too weak to even handle this device. Eventually, I took the easy way out and grew a beard and mustache, much to the dismay of my wife. I finally, though, convinced her that my beard would make her life easier as well since she would only need to trim it occasionally rather than shave me daily.

My ability to comb and brush my hair also decreased as my arm strength weakened. However, figure 18 shows long-handled brushes and combs that are adjustable and lock at any desired angle. These helped me tremendously.

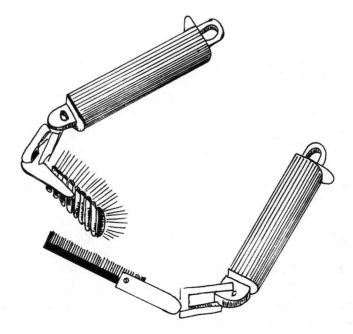

Figure 18 Long-Handled Brush and Comb

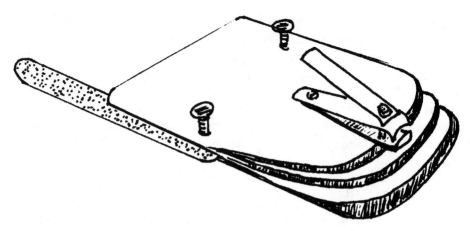

Figure 19 Nail Clipper

The nail clipper/file board shown in figure 19 provides one-handed ease in clipping fingernails. The suction-cup base holds the platform in place on any smooth flat surface and the long levered clipper trims nails easily. The nail clipper also contains side slots to mount emery boards.

SITTING, STANDING, AND MOBILITY AIDS

Sitting Aids

As my legs and hip muscles deteriorated, it became harder for me to rise from a sitting position. For a while, I was limited to sitting in straight-backed wooden chairs or forced to ask for assistance every time I needed to get up from a recliner, deep-seated sofa, or a soft-cushioned chair. However, I soon alleviated this problem by setting my recliner on a five-inch platform and by extending the legs of a chair by five inches (figure 20). Leg extenders can add three to five inches to the height of any chair or bed with straight legs. These devices do not cause any damage to the user's furniture and can be used for either temporary or permanent use.

One device I purchased was a lifter seat (figure 20), which is advertised to "raise you like magic—with very little effort." The seat is essentially a 16-inch by 4-inch cushion designed to gently raise users as they lean forward in their chairs. However, I found that the lifter seat is quite expensive, uncomfortable, and failed to raise me high enough to stand without any assistance. However, an individual whose disability has stabilized may want to invest in a recliner chair that has a permanent built-in mechanism.

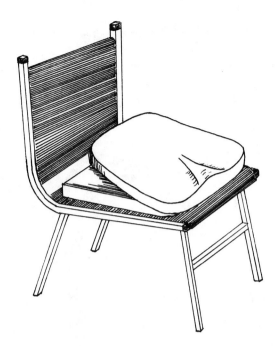

Figure 20   Lifter Seat

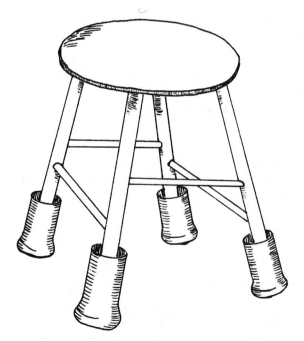

Figure 21   Leg Extenders

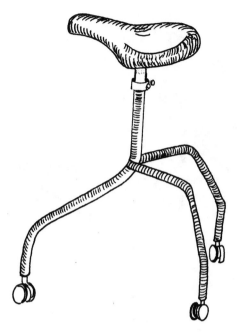

Figure 22 Rolling Stool

Standing Aids

The three-legged rolling stool shown in figure 22 allows an individual's back, legs, and feet to rest while he/she continues to "stand." This mobile stool supports nearly 90 percent of body weight, enabling the user to enjoy the comforts of sitting while in a near-standing position. It may also be raised from 24 to 34 inches.

A roll-around cart, similar to a butler's cart or a small shopping basket, is ideal for carrying things around the house, such as laundry, groceries, and cleaning supplies. It also serves as a modified "walker" that provides the user with support while moving around.

Mobility Aids

Canes

One of the first mobility devices I obtained was a cane. After much resistance, I finally listened to my physical therapist who suggested that I use a cane to help me walk more steadily and easily. When my wife witnessed me walking with a cane for the first time, she commented on how much more steadily I was moving around. A cane enhances the safety and stability of walking by providing additional support. The use of a cane, however, requires moderate strength in

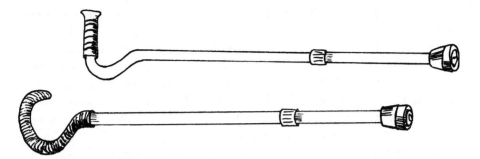

Figure 23 Canes with horizontal handles

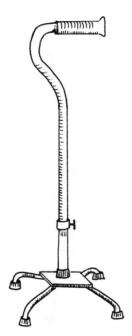

Figure 24 Quad Cane

the user's hands and arms. A cane may be most useful when one leg is significantly weaker than the other, as mine were. The recommended method is to hold the cane on the side of the good leg. Since my right leg was weaker than my left one, I held the cane in my left hand. This procedure allows some of the body weight to shift away from the weaker side of the body and allows a wider base of support. With only a few minutes of instruction and practice, the pattern of my walking became smooth and natural. My physical therapist stressed that if I purchased another cane to buy one with a height suited for me. In other words, one with which the top of the cane is aligned with my wrist. This allows for a proper elbow-angle bend when the cane is in use.

Canes come in a number of different styles—each contoured to the strength of the user's hands and shoulders. For example, figure 23 displays a cane with a horizontal grip and one with a hook grip. The horizontal-grip cane supplies a more secure grip for a person with a weak hand because the horizontal handle provides a greater weight-bearing surface for the user's hand. The "Quad" cane shown in figure 24 has four feet; this design provides more stability than a straight cane. The major disadvantage with this multi-footed cane is the additional weight that must be manipulated by the user. Even with the advent of lighter-weight materials and high-impact plastics, the weight of the Quad cane is often double that of the straight cane.

Crutches

Since my arm and shoulder muscles were weak, my physical therapist advised me not to use an armpit-type (auxiliary) crutch. However, for those who do have sufficient arm and shoulder strength I recommend the "Canadian" crutch. Again, patients should work closely with their physical therapists when selecting crutches.

Walkers

About ten months after I began using my cane, I found that walking any significant distance was both exhausting and risky. As a result, my physical therapist suggested that I use a walker. Since my local medical supply store allowed customers to rent walkers on a monthly, trial basis, I was able to try a number of different walkers before purchasing one. Monthly rental fees were then deducted from the final purchase price. Those who are interested in walkers should check their local medical suppliers for similar opportunities to preview equipment.

To operate a walker, individuals must have moderate strength in their hands and arms. As with a cane, finding a walker that fits the user appropriately is important. The walker's hand grip should be leveled to the user's wrist when it is relaxed at his or her side. A standard walker (figure 25) requires enough arm strength to lift and move the walker with each step. A rolling walker (figure 26) contains front-wheeled attachments which allow the user to push instead of lift the walker. The rolling walker, however, is a less stable device than the regular walker. For more control, users may add spring-loaded brakes to the walker's rear legs. I discovered that in addition to the wheels and brakes, it was important for me to have a walker that could easily be folded and transported in a car. Figure 26 also shows a walker with armrests which may be used by individuals who have insufficient arm strength but adequate shoulder strength to support their own weight.

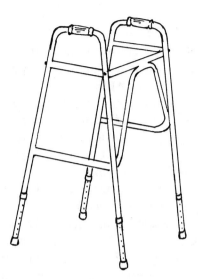

Figure 25   Standard Walker

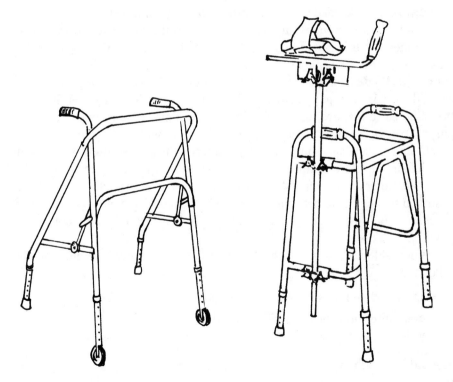

Figure 26   Walkers with modifications

Wheelchairs

"Excessive fatigue, unsteadiness, difficulty rising from a chair, and occasional falls are indications that you are in need of more support than that provided by your present mobility aids."[1] I began to experience all of these symptoms about one year after my diagnosis. However, like most people needing a wheelchair, I was reluctant to even talk about needing this device because I felt that in doing so I was surrendering to my disease. Although I had looked at electric scooters as a possible solution since they didn't "look" like wheelchairs, I still viewed any type of wheeled assistance as my enemy.

I was soon forced to re-examine the wheelchair issue when I collapsed during a business meeting. I had parked my car about 100 yards from the building where the meeting was to be held. By the time I arrived at the building, my legs were wobbly and weak. Soon thereafter, my legs completely gave out as I entered the lobby of the building, and I ended up falling on my head. Although I didn't suffer any physical injuries, I did suffer from humiliation. This incident was certainly a wake-up call, and I was forced to decide whether I wanted to continue working and use a wheelchair or stop working altogether. Since I enjoyed working, I decided that it was time to purchase a wheelchair.

A wheelchair provides an interface between the disabled and the world around them. In the United States today there are hundreds of companies that make thousands of wheelchairs and scooters. With so many design factors and options to choose from, selecting a wheelchair can be a bewildering experience as well as a very expensive task. Although all wheelchairs generally have the same basic features, the mechanisms controlling these features vary. The purpose of this section is not to provide readers with a complete guide to purchasing wheelchairs, but to provide readers with general information about wheelchairs and to describe some of the various types of wheeled mobility available. Refer to Chapter 4, "Sources of Equipment and Supplies," for wheelchair and scooter manufacturing sources. The final decision on which model to purchase should be made by the patient, his or her doctor, and the consulting physical therapist.

When selecting a wheelchair to purchase, individuals should do the following:

- Decide what kind of assistance is required
- Determine how the chair will be used

Manual Wheelchairs

When considering which type of assistance is necessary, individuals must ascertain what kinds of activity they are able to do considering the level and degree of their physical impairment. For example, those with strong upper-body muscles

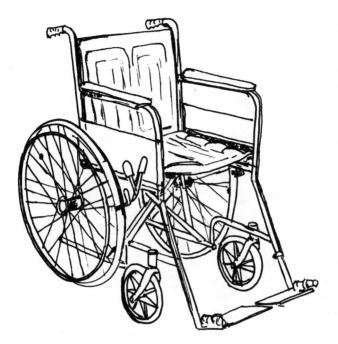

Figure 27   Standard Wheelchair

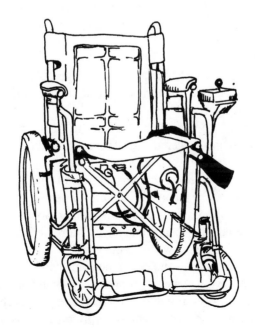

Figure 28   Traditional-Style Electric Wheelchair

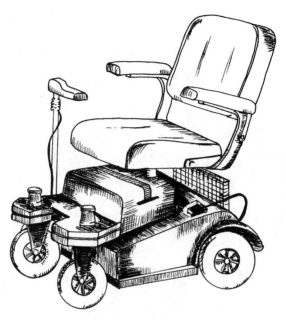

Figure 29 Platform-Model Powered Chair

can operate a manual wheelchair that is propelled by arm strength. There are a variety of manual wheelchairs available, including high-speed racing models. Figure 27 displays a standard manual wheelchair. However, individuals with weak upper-arm strength and weak leg strength should use a powered chair.

Powered Wheelchairs

The traditional powered wheelchair, as shown in figure 28, is similar to a manual chair except that it has added batteries and added control mechanisms to support the additional weight.

The platform-model powered chair, shown in figure 29, consists of a seating platform mounted on a powered base. This type of wheelchair contains many variations and options to choose from.

The three- and four-wheeled scooters, shown in figures 30 and 31, respectively, are alternatives to the manual or powered wheelchair. Scooters provide a form of mobility that does not look like a wheelchair. Scooters are not as expensive as regular powered wheelchairs and have a narrower wheelbase that is usually more maneuverable than a wheelchair.

It is also important to determine how the chair will be used. For instance, I wanted to be able to use my power chair both indoors and outdoors—on smooth paved surfaces as well as on rough grass. I also preferred a chair that could be easily transported since I hoped to continue my business activities as long as possible. Lastly, I wanted the chair to be flexible enough to last throughout my

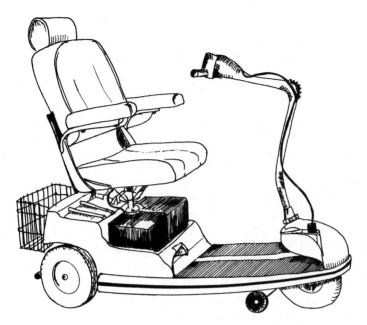

Figure 30 Three-Wheeled Scooter

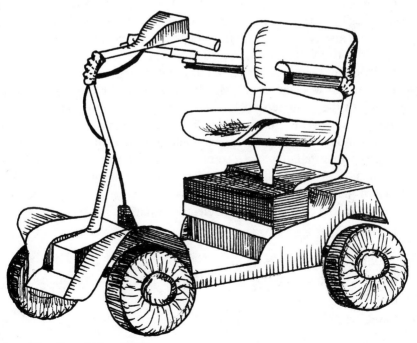

Figure 31 Four-Wheeled Scooter

entire disability. As my level of dependency increases, I need a chair that will continue to adjust to my circumstances and remain suitable for me.

After considering all of these factors, I purchased a scooter that could be converted from a three-wheeled model to a four-wheeled model. The steering mechanism on the three-wheeled model is similar to the handlebars on a bicycle, while the four-wheeled model contains a steering mechanism similar to a tiller. With a removable seat, both versions of the scooter can be easily transported into the rear compartment of a small station wagon. With the addition of a small electric hoist installed in the wagon, the scooter can be loaded and unloaded in less than five minutes.

For several months while I was still able to drive, I continued to maintain my independence with very little inconvenience. However, now I am no longer able to drive or use my hands and arms effectively. As a result, I have converted the tiller on the four-wheeled model to a joystick that I can operate with just my thumb and forefinger. In the future, I will probably add a highback seat and a headrest to the scooter.

I have discovered certain advantages to using a scooter. First of all, the scooter which I operate has an electric-powered seat which can be raised and lowered by five inches. This device enables me to be raised up to almost a standing position, making it easy to transfer from the scooter to another chair or to use the restroom. Secondly, the scooter has a powerful motor which allows it to climb ramps that are considerably shorter than what is needed for a manual wheelchair. For instance, I am able to go up a 25-degree ramp, or one with a four-foot run and a one-foot rise. In comparison, a manual wheelchair requires a ramp with a twelve-foot run and a one-foot rise.

Two kinds of ramps are available for wheeled-assistance users: metal fabricated ramps and wooden ramps. Metal ramps, however, are quite expensive. The length of the ramp depends on both the total height of the stairs and the slope of the ramp. A low guardrail should run the length of the ramp to prevent users from rolling off. I found that a one-inch-high lip on the edge of the ramp is effective as a guardrail. It is also recommended that long ramps have at least one handrail that is 30 to 32 inches high. If the entry level of a user's residence is so high that it makes using a ramp impractical (by being too steep or too long), individuals should consider using an electric porch lift. A typical unit is shown in figure 32.

Wheelchair Accessories

Here are a few of the many accessories that can be obtained for almost any type wheelchair:

Trays

Lapboard

Worktables

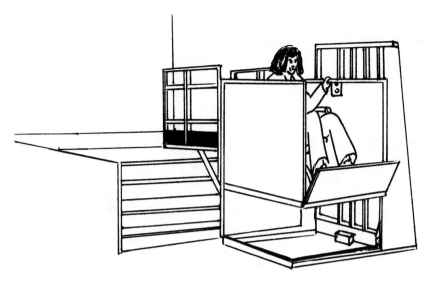

Figure 32   Porch Lift

Arm Slings

Heel and Toe Loops

Heel Strap

Storage Pocket

Crutch and Cane Holder

Removable Headrest

Head Wings

Adjustable Footrest

Wrist Cuffs

Foam Seats

Inflatable Rubber Cushion

Safety Straps

Wheelchair manufacturers can supply these accessories as well as many more (refer to Chapter 4, "Sources of Equipment and Supplies"). Custom orders are also available, however, they are both expensive and usually take a lengthy period to receive.

Road Vehicles

My experience with road vehicles is very limited. As I lost arm and hand strength and dexterity, I considered modifying my vehicle to allow me to continue to drive. However, the progression of my disease accelerated and it soon became evident that I would only be able to drive for a short period of time at best. As a result, I dropped the idea since I wouldn't want a driver like myself on the road under any condition. Refer to Chapter 4, "Sources of Equipment and Supplies," for vehicle-modification sources.

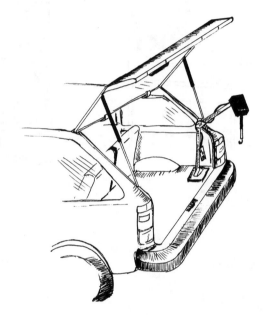

Figure 33   Electric Hoist mounted in station wagon

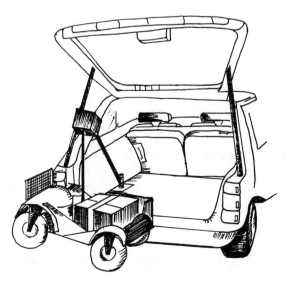

Figure 34   Scooter on Hoist

However, what I did do was modify my station wagon in a way that allowed me to easily transport my electric scooter. Figures 33, 34, 35, and 36 display how an electric hoist was mounted at the rear of the wagon's tailgate. With the assistance of the electric hoist, it now takes approximately three to four minutes to load the scooter into the rear of the wagon.

While the electric hoist in our situation is permanently mounted, figure 34 shows how this same hoist can be mounted in a portable, temporary manner so that it can be used in the trunk of a standard sedan.

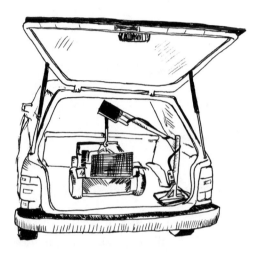

Figure 35 Scooter in station wagon

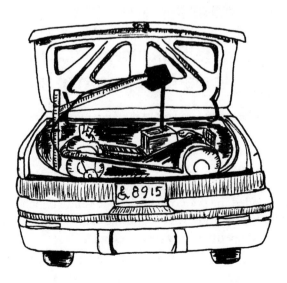

Figure 36 Scooter in trunk of sedan

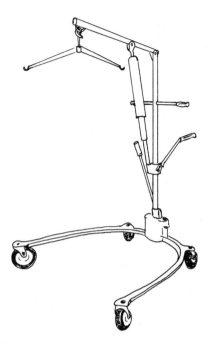

Figure 37   Hydraulic Lifter

Another mobility aid is the mechanical or hydraulic lifter. This type of lifter allows a person to transfer a totally dependent patient with ease. This device is especially useful in situations where the patient is larger than the caregiver. The hydraulic lifter is generally considered easier to operate since it features caster wheels and an adjustable base for easy positioning.

HOME FURNISHINGS AND HOME MODIFICATIONS

As I grew more house-bound and more dependent on my power chair, I realized that movement around my house could be made easier with a few minor modifications. For instance, with the construction of ramps, I was not only able to move freely inside my house, but I could enter and leave it independently as well. Special hinges were also installed enabling doors to open flat against the wall and thus extended the door openings by about two inches (figure 38). This addition has enabled me to move around the house with my scooter, which is about 25 inches wide, without any inconvenience.

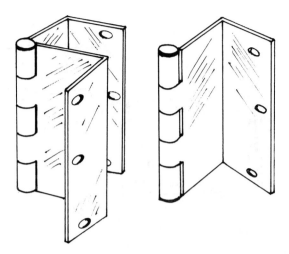

Figure 38   Special Flush Hinges

Those who want to get from one floor to another without any assistance many want to purchase a stair lift. The one that I obtained was simple to install and is leased on a yearly basis.

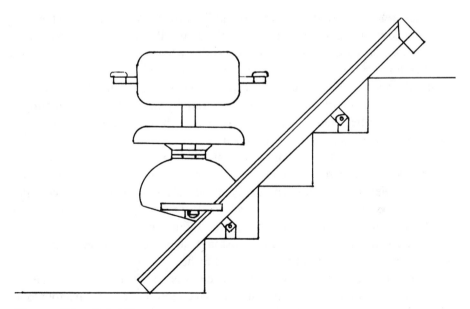

Figure 39   Stair Lift

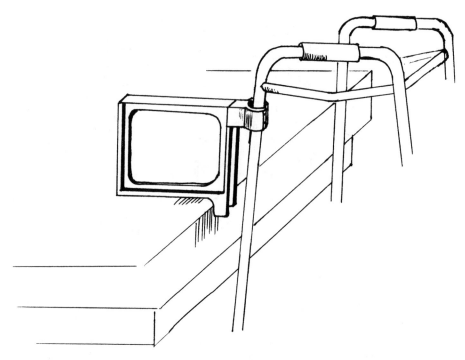

Figure 40   Assist Handle

There are many additional devices and fixtures available that make the goal of independent living more attainable. For example, the Assist Handle feature in figure 40 assists patients in rising from a sitting position to a standing position. The handle attaches to a walker and rotates to rest on the surface of a bed or chair. Patients may then simply push down on the handle and lift themselves up.

Another version of this device is shown in figure 41. The bed rail simply attaches to any bed frame and assists patients with positioning themselves in bed as well as getting into and out of bed.

Where permanent living modifications are too expensive or impractical, all-purpose devices such as the bedside commode chair shown in figure 42 are affordable. This type of unit can be used as one of the following: a raised toilet seat with safety rails, a free-standing commode, or a bath and shower seat. This unit comes with a splash guard for use over a toilet, and with a fitted pail so it can be used anywhere in the home. Most units also come with adjustable legs that can raise the seat height from 18 to 22 inches.

Two other inexpensive devices are the leg lifter and the rope ladder. The leg lifter is about 42 inches long and contains a hand loop at one end and a foot loop at the other end. This device assists users in raising and lowering their legs from a bed or wheelchair.

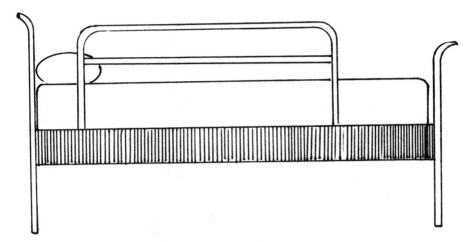

Figure 41   Bed Rail

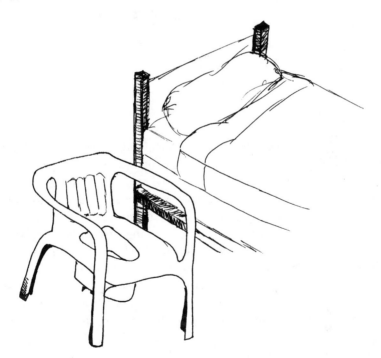

Figure 42   Bedside Commode

The rope ladder (see figure 43) is ideal for people who have difficulty sitting up in bed. The rope ladder has wide rungs that users with minimal arm and hand strength can grab onto hand-over-hand, while rising to a sitting position.

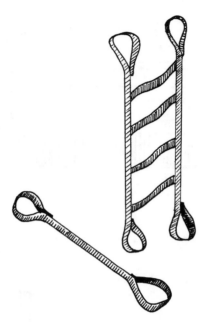

Figure 43   Rope Ladder and Leg Lifter

Household Tips

Many people who are confined to a wheelchair face everyday household restrictions and barriers. The normal height of a light switch from a floor, for instance, may be too high for an individual in a wheelchair who has weak arm and shoulder muscles. Fortunately, there is a wide variety of adaptations and modifications available that help promote independence and safety. As indicated in the previous section, these modifications range from the very simple and inexpensive to the very complex and costly. Each individual must assess their own needs and decide what, if any, changes are necessary and practical.

I found that since my condition changed frequently, what had worked at one time was not sufficient at another time. It was therefore necessary for me to weigh the costs of a modification against the length of time it would be useful. Many things that may have eased my daily living for a relatively short period of time were too costly and too impractical for me to purchase.

Listed below are household tips for increasing accessibility within the household:

- Doorsills should be removed whenever possible.
- Throw rugs and thick carpeting should be avoided.
- Use nonskid floors.
- Furniture should be arranged appropriately to allow traffic access.

- Doors should be eliminated when possible and changed to either sliding or folding doors, or curtains.
- Bathing and toilet facilities should be outfitted with grab bars and non-skid flooring.
- A communication system should be within reach and of a type usable by the patient.
- Ideally doorways should be 32 to 34 inches wide.
- Beds should have 36 inches of space on three sides.
- Long leverfaucets can replace standard faucets for easier reach.
- A kickplate can be mounted at the base of a door to prevent marring the wood when the footrest of the wheelchair is used to push the door open.
- An extension switch can be installed over an existing switch allowing a person otherwise unable to reach the switch to control the lights.
- Environmental control centers are available which allow an individual to control lights, television, radio, and even answer a phone from an easily transportable remote control.

Kitchen Aids

I consider myself fortunate that my wife is available to prepare all of my meals. Because of this, I do not have to fend for myself in the kitchen. I am familiar, though, with kitchen tools and utensils and, at times, have enjoyed being able to prepare and serve a wide variety of foods myself. I discovered a number of assistive devices by thumbing through several catalogs devoted to independent living. For example, one-handed easy-to-use peelers, graters, choppers, and so on, are available. Electric blenders, meat grinders, juicers, and mixers all make food preparation easier and more convenient. Safety devices are also available, such as long matches, push-button fire extinguishers, and stove guards. These devices provide peace of mind not only to the person working in the kitchen, but to those who are depending on the kitchen user to be careful. Metal tongs, long-handled bottle and can openers, lid flippers, vise-type jar openers, clamps, and other holders are also available for one-handed kitchen work.

Cleaning Aids

Some assistive devices for cleaning and routine maintenance include long-handled dusters and dust pans, high-handled wet mops, lightweight vacuum cleaners; and all-purpose tongs. Also available are long-handled bathtub scrubbers and sponges, sink mats to reduce breakage, suction-based brushes for kitchen counters, lightweight irons, and adjustable ironing boards that can even fit across the arms of a wheelchair.

Reading, Writing, and Communication Aids

One of my favorite leisure activities has always been reading. As my other activities diminished due to loss of strength, I resorted to reading everything and anything I could get my hands on. But when my hands and arms began to fail, holding a book and turning its pages also became difficult for me to do. However, this was easily resolved by obtaining a book rack like the one shown in figure 44. Book racks are available in many different sizes and designs.

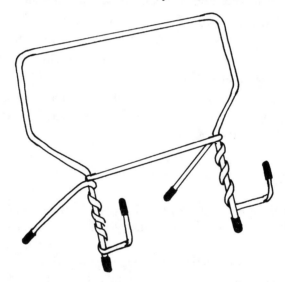

Figure 44 Book Rack

Individuals who are confined to a bed may find overhead book holders with automatic page turners extremely useful. Also available are prismatic glasses for prone reading, as shown in figure 45. Glasses of this type enable people to read or watch television while lying flat. The prism turns the image to a right angle so no head movement is necessary to view the image. Nonautomatic page turners, such as rubber-tipped sticks or thimbles, sticks with magnets, and mouth sticks with suction cups all provide hands-free assistance for patients whose mouths and jaws are strong enough to hold the device. Other devices that are worth considering by persons confined to their beds are microfilmed books read with ceiling or wall projectors, and books on audiocassette.

Pens given to arthritis sufferers are useful. Pens similar to the one shown in figure 46 are designed so that almost no pressure is required to use the pen. This pen also has a slight indentation in the thumb area for an easy grip.

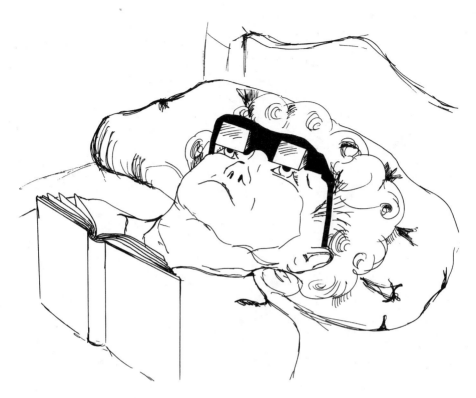

Figure 45   Prism Glasses

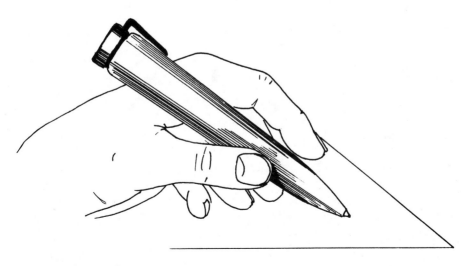

Figure 46   Flat Pen

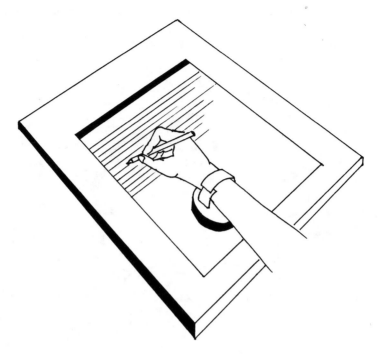

Figure 47   Magnetized Writing Board

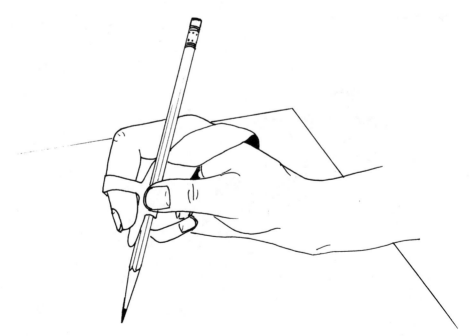

Figure 48   Writing Cuff

For sufferers of cerebral palsy, Parkinson's disease, or mild hand tremors, magnetized writing boards used for holding paper (figure 47) are available. This device features a magnetic holder that users can fasten onto their wrists with Velcro straps.

Finger pen holders are ideal for arthritic and stroke patients who have some hand movement but have limited or weak grasping abilities. This writing cuff has a small pen attached to a band which slips over the user's index finger. In addition, customized writing aids like the one shown in figure 48 provide persons with decreased dexterity the ability to hold their fingers in a proper position.

Communication Devices

Individuals who suffer nerve damage as a result of an accident, stroke, or injuries to the nerve muscles may experience speech problems. Patients who have good use of their hands and arms may use writing and gestures as forms of communication to replace speech for at least some messages. Patients who have lost the manual dexterity necessary for writing can communicate by typing on a computer or typewriter-style keyboard. Since there are a great many communication aids available, I will not attempt to list them all here, but instead only describe a few examples. Keep in mind that with the rapid advance of electronic technology, even the examples described here are quickly becoming obsolete with the development of smaller and faster "message transmitters." Communication aids are arbitrarily divided into two main groups: "message transmitters" and "communication boards."

People with diminished voice volume may be able to use a small amplifier. This device which is held in the hand or placed around the neck amplifies the speaker's voice through a detached speaker. The amplifier, however, is generally not helpful for persons who experience difficulty in forming words. Those who have a weak voice because their vocal cords are not vibrating normally may use an electrolarynx. This device is an artificial voice source; it creates a robot-like sound which the user can turn into words by pressing the device against the throat.

Voice Synthesizers

Every morning in Africa, a gazelle wakes up.
It knows that it must run faster than the fastest lion,
Or it will be killed.
Every morning in Africa, a lion wakes up.
It knows that it must outrun the slowest gazelle,
Or it will starve to death.
It doesn't matter whether you're a lion or a gazelle.
When the sun comes up in the morning, you'd better be running!

This poem was featured in an article titled, "Eyes on the Prize" in *PC Magazine.*[2]

According to the article, the poem was written by a man who is completely paralyzed and is dying of ALS. He was able to write the poem on a personal computer by wearing a pair of infrared sensor glasses and by blinking his eyelids.

This individual's personal computer was provided to him by a group known as "Voice for Joanie." This program provides computer voice synthesizers to people who have lost their ability to speak. With corporate donations from IBM, Microsoft, the Connecticut Union of Telecommunication Workers, and many other private groups and individuals, Voice for Joanie has placed more than 87 systems in 66 Connecticut towns since 1990 and has helped many disabled men and women regain their ability to communicate. Voice for Joanie was started by Shirley Fredlund, a friend of Joan Margaitis who was paralyzed with ALS and was not able to speak. Shirley searched for the technology that could give Joanie her voice back. One year later, the computer program was fully developed. Unfortunately, Joanie Margaitis died a few days before it was ready for her to use.

The communicator created by Voice for Joanie consists of a personal computer equipped with special software, a voice synthesizer, an infra-red eye switch, and a printer. If a person is able to blink, nod or move a finger, he or she will be able to "speak" by highlighting the words or phrases on the screen of the computer. The built-in synthesizer then translates the words into speech. This equipment is usually loaned to patients for as long as they need to communicate.

For more information regarding the Voice for Joanie program, write or call:

Voice for Joanie
49 East Street
New Milford, CT 06776
(203) 355-2611, Ext. 4517

Voice-Activated Computer Systems

As I continued to deteriorate physically, I found that it became more and more difficult for me to communicate by keyboarding messages. The Voice for Joanie program informed me of a computer program available known as DragonDictate. Essentially, the DragonDictate dictation system recognizes what is said by the speaker and matches the spoken words against its built-in set of vocabulary words. There are three levels of DragonDictate Systems available:

DragonDictate Starter Edition	Contains a vocabulary of 5,000 words. This program is designed for users who create

documents on specific topics and for those who need an efficient alternate to their keyboards.

DragonDictate Classic Edition
This edition contains a vocabulary of 30,000 words. It is designed for users whose work requires a large and versatile vocabulary.

DragonDictate

Power Edition
As of mid-1994, this is the most powerful speech-recognition program available. It has a 60,000-active-word vocabulary and is designed for professionals whose work requires an extensive, specialized, or technical vocabulary.

The computer system needed to run DragonDictate consists of:

- 486/33 personal computer
- MS-DOS 5.0 or later
- 3.5-inch high-density diskette drive
- 8 MB RAM for the Starter Edition; 12 MB RAM for the Classic Edition; and, 16 MB RAM for the Power Edition
- 31 MB of hard disk space for the Starter Edition; 37 MB for the Classic Edition; and, 46 MB for the Power Edition
- EISA/ISA or MCA slot for a speech board

About three weeks after I obtained a DragonDictate program, I was able to dictate 35 to 40 words per minute. For more information regarding DragonDictate write to the following address:

Dragon Systems
320 Nevada Street
Newton, MA 02160
(800) 825-5897

In addition to DragonDictate, two other similar software programs are available: IBM VoiceType Dictation for OS/2 and Kurzwell Voice 1.0 for Windows. For more information on these two programs please call:

IBM VoiceType Dictation for OS/2
(800) 825-5263
Kurzwell Voice 1.0 for Windows
Kurzwell Applied Intelligence
(800) 380-1234

Communication Boards

To some extent, the voice synthesizer is, in fact a "communication board," in the sense that a message is created on a screen by an artificially created voice. Communication boards, however, are usually devices that both the patient and the listener can use to communicate. These boards are typically used by severely paralyzed patients who are able to transmit messages by using eye movement rather than other muscular motions.

There are several types of communication boards available, but all are generally used in the same manner. The board is set up in a place where the patient and the listener can clearly see the board and each other. The patient transmits a message by pointing to or looking at symbols on the board. The listener then relays back to the patient the message he/she thinks is being sent. With practice, both the patient and the listener can become very adept at using the board. One example of a communication board is the "Etran" (figure 49). The Etran consists of a transparent board with letters and numbers arranged in groups. Words are spelled out by looking at the places on the board where the letters and numbers are located.

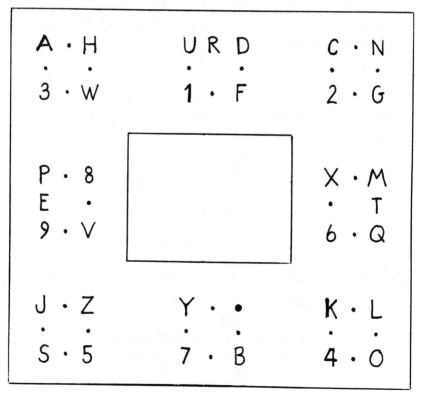

Figure 49   The Etran Board

Telephone Aids

When the ability for me to readily get up and answer a phone was greatly reduced, I purchased a portable phone which I kept beside me on my power chair. However, when the weakness in my hands and arms prevented me from even handling a light portable phone, I purchased a speakerphone. To dial and operate the phone I use a mouth stick with a rubber tip. Dialing was also made easier with the use of programmable numbers and automated dialing.

Other options users may want to consider are the shoulder rest and the swing-away receiver. The shoulder rest, which can be purchased at any stationery or office supply store, enables the user to have a hands-free telephone conversation. The swing-away receiver consists of a holding bracket with an easily reachable off/on switch which also provides a hands-free setup.

Emergency Aids

One extremely lightweight device that I carry on my power scooter all the time is a cellular phone. This device enables me to immediately alert my caregiver in the case of an emergency. It weighs a mere 7.2 ounces and can be carried in my shirt pocket.

Disabled persons may also want to invest in various alert systems. Alert systems typically consist of a small pendant that users wear around their necks. These systems are easy to install and cost between $100 and $400.

When the button on the pendant is pushed, an automatic dialer is activated and dials up to five numbers in sequence until someone answers. On the receiving end of the emergency call, a recorded message of the user's voice is heard. For example the listener may hear the following message: "There's an emergency at my house. Press zero to listen in. If you don't hear me, call for help immediately." When the listeners press the zero key, they are confirming that they received the call and have activated the listen-in feature.

Disabled persons may also wish to connect to a professional monitoring service. A monitored console uses a digital communicator instead of a pre-recorded voice message. When activated by the pendant, the console dials the response center's computer and transmits a unique identification code. Within a few seconds, an attendant is able to access the user's medical history, list of response people and agencies, as well as the user's address directions. Some consoles also supply a two-way voice communicator, greatly improving the odds that an attendant can make contact with the user in case of an actual emergency.

National monitoring centers typically charge up to $45 a month. The monitoring devices are usually leased rather than sold, and therefore the total monthly charge is considerably higher. Prices vary dramatically, so shop around. Several companies that manufacture monitored and unmonitored personal emergency response systems are listed in Chapter 4 under "Personal Emergency-Response

Systems." The list includes toll-free phone numbers and a brief description of each system.

My search for devices that will improve my daily living is endless. In fact, I have just begun to search for an electric, hospital-type bed. Since I am beginning to experience difficulty in breathing at night, the adjustable bed will allow me to raise my head and ease my breathing.

Since there are hundreds of manual and electronic devices available to make daily living easier, I found that the easiest way to keep abreast of all of these products is to request catalogs from supply companies. Refer to the following chapter for my complete listing of suppliers. Additionally, your occupational or physical therapist has access to many catalogs.

One last point I want to emphasize is that disabled persons must learn to take control of their lives. Although caregivers and others may assist, it is really up to them to maintain some kind of independent living.

Sources of Equipment and Supplies

The following are companies that supply general and specialized assistive devices and equipment. Since new companies and products are emerging on a daily basis, any attempt to provide an updated listing would be futile. However, the companies listed in this section will give users a starting point.

The products and descriptions listed in the following pages are for informational purposes only. I have not personally examined or tested all of these products, and I do not endorse or represent them.

For additional company and product listings, refer to the *Thomas Register*, a commercial publication that lists thousands of companies by product type and category. The *Thomas Register* can be found in most public libraries. In addition to the *Thomas Register*, caregivers and individuals with disabilities can easily tap into a wide range of assistive device resources through a service called ABLEDATA—a service provided by the National Rehabilitation Information Center. ABLEDATA is a database that contains an extensive listing of nearly 20,000 assistive devices available from national and international sources. Each listing includes the product's price and a brief description. To find out more about ABLEDATA, contact the ABLEDATA staff at:

- ABLEDATA, 8455 Colesville Road, Suite 935, Silver Spring, MD 20910; (800) 227-0216 or (301) 588-9284; fax (301) 587-1967 (Hours of service are 8 a.m. to 6 p.m. Eastern time, Monday through Friday except Federal holidays.)
- ABLE INFORM BBS (Bulletin Board Service). This service is also available 24 hours a day. It is accessible to patrons with a computer, modem, and telecommunications software and provides access to the

ABLEDATA database and the NARIC databases on disability and rehabilitation literature and resources. ABLE INFORM BBS also provides conferencing, bulletins, and classified listings of previously owned assistive and adaptive devices. Experienced BBS users can call (301) 589-3563 (line settings of 1200 to 9600 baud, N-8-1). First-time or novice users are encouraged to call the office for a brochure.

- CD-ROM version of the ABLEDATA database may be purchased for use on your own computer. Release dates are March and September; updates between releases are available on the ABLE INFORM BBS and on diskette. Contact the information specialist at (800) 227-0216 to obtain a detailed brochure of this option.

The following list of medical devices and equipment suppliers is just a sampling of supplier information that I have obtained during my search for acceptable daily living aids. Some selections originated from the ABLEDATA database. Some of these listings offer sample products.

GENERAL MEDICAL DEVICES AND EQUIPMENT

American Hospital Supply Company, 6600 West Touhy Avenue, Chicago, IL 60648; (804) 424-5200

Adaptability, Post Office Box 515, Colchester, CT 06415-0515; (800) 288-9941

Cleo Living Aids, 3957 Mayfield Road, Cleveland, OH 44121; (216) 382-9700 or (800) 321-0595

Guardian Products, a Division of Sunrise Medical, 4175 Guardian Street, Simi Valley, CA 93063; (800) 255-5022

MOBILITY PRODUCTS: Walkers, canes, crutches, and manual wheelchairs.

BATHROOM SAFETY EQUIPMENT: Bath seats, transfer benches, hand-held showers, toilet safety frames, three-in-one commodes, rolling commodes, transport commodes, grab bars, and safety rails.

PATIENT HANDLING EQUIPMENT: Hydraulic, crank and electric patient hoists, bathtub lifters, pool lifters, and auto transfer hoists.

Invacare Corporation, 899 Cleveland Street, Elyria, OH 44035; (800) 333-6900

MOBILITY PRODUCTS: Canes, crutches, walkers, manual and electric wheelchairs.

MOBILITE HEALTH CARE BEDS: Electrically operated health care beds, semi-electric health care beds (head and foot adjustment electric, up and down manual crank), manually operated beds.

PORTABLE PATIENT LIFTS: Hydraulic lifts limited to a capacity of 450 pounds; crank lift limit 300 pounds. Masts are interchangeable with bases. Optional bases include C, U, and offset. Five-inch casters on all bases designs. A variety of sling designs in canvas or nylon mesh are available.

BATH SAFETY EQUIPMENT: Bathtub transfer benches, shower and tub benches, hand-held showers, grab bars, bedside commodes, and three-in-one commodes.

Lumex, Incorporated, 100 Spence Street, Bay Shore, NY 11706-2290; (516) 273-2200 or (800) 645-5272

BATHROOM SAFETY EQUIPMENT: Grab bars and bathtub safety rails, bath seats, transfer tub benches, hand-held showers, toilet safety frames, raised seats and accessories, three-in-one commodes, transport commodes, and commode chairs.

MOBILITY PRODUCTS: Canes, walkers, and crutches, manual wheelchairs.

PATIENT ROOM EQUIPMENT: Trapezes, bedrails, bed tables, IV stands, hampers, bags, carts and accessories.

PRESSURE MANAGEMENT: Pressure-reduction mattresses and pressure-management cushions.

HOME CARE SEATING: Rockers and recliners.

Maddak, Incorporated, 6 Industrial Road, Pequannock, NJ 07440; (201) 628-7600 or (800) 443-4926

Fred Sammons/Enrichments, Post Office Box 471, Western Springs, IL 60558-0471; (800) 323-5547

GENERAL DAILY LIVING PRODUCTS: Exercise products, arthritic/massage, daily living products, kitchen and dining aids, nutrition products, diabetic care products, seating and tables, bedroom accessories, mobility assists, wheelchair accessories, back supports, quick change clothing and other dressing aids, incontinence products, skin and wound care, bathroom and grooming products.

AIDS FOR THE BLIND AND VISUALLY HANDICAPPED

American Foundation for the Blind, 15 West 16th Street, New York, NY 10011; (212) 620-2175

LEATHER COIN PURSE/KEY HOLDER: This leather coin purse/ key holder is an organized and secure means of holding up to four quarters, eight dimes, four nickels, and six pennies. This black purse also has a pocket for paper money and six hook key holders. It measures $2^{1}/_{2}$ by $3^{5}/_{8}$ inches.

American Printing House for the Blind, 1839 Frankfort Avenue, Louisville, KY 40206; (502) 895-2405

WOODEN BRAILLE ERASER: The wooden Braille eraser is made of maple with a natural finish. It has a round tip on one end and on the other a handle with a flattened side to prevent the eraser from rolling away. It measures $2^{1}/_{2}$ inches long.

CORRECTING SLATES AND STYLUSES: The correcting slates and styluses are designed for correcting Braille by allowing for the addition of missing dots on sheets of Braille up to $11^{1}/_{2}$ inches wide. The slates are made of metal and have 38 cells per line. Two versions are available: one has pins which can also be used as a regular slate (1–00190–00); the other does not have pins (1–00130–00). Both measure $11^{1}/_{4}$ by $1^{3}/_{4}$ inches.

AUTOMOBILE OPTIONS AND RESOURCES

Anafield Corporation, 3219 West Washington, Indianapolis, IN 46222; (317) 636-8061

> Remote Control Starter: Remote Start is a radio remote control for an automobile starter. It can determine hot or cold start procedures and restarts automatically if the engine stalls. It has a safety shutdown to prevent battery drain if the vehicle will not start. The radio transmitter has a 100-foot range.

American Automobile Manufacturer's Association, 1401 H Street NW, Washington, DC 20015; (202) 326-5500

The Chrysler Motors Physically Challenged Resource Center, Post Office Box 159, Detroit, MI 48288-0159; (800) 255-9877

Handicaps Incorporated, 4335 South Santa Fe Drive, Englewood, CO 80110; (303) 781-2062

> HAND BRAKE/CLUTCH CONTROL: The Hand Brake/Clutch Control is a hand clutch control designed for people who are unable to use their left leg.

The Department of Transportation, 400 Seventh Street SW, Washington, DC 20591; (202) 366-4000 or (800) 424-9393; TDD (202) 755-8919 or TDD (800) 424-9153

Meyra Incorporated, 59 Wedgewood Road, Newark, DE 19711-2055; (302) 324-4400 or (800) 833-9962

> CAR LIFTER: This transfer lift for cars has a sideways swiveling lifter suspended on a mast installed between the vehicle floor and instrument panel. A second swivel axle provides adjustment variations. Height adjustable by an electric motor connected to car's 12-volt battery with a control box containing a switch for verticle movement fastened to cable for attendant or user operation. Attaches via magnetic disc. Lifter may be removed from mast or swiveled and stored beside the door. This aid may be used on driver or passenger side of car, and is made of black plastic-coated metal parts with a mesh fabric seat. Maximum load capacity is approximately 220 pounds.

Mobility Products and Design, 14800 28th Avenue North, Minneapolis, MN 55447; (612) 559-1680 or (800) 488-7688

HAND CONTROL: The Hand Control is designed for persons without the use of their left leg to operate the brake pedal or clutch. This lightweight brushed aluminum alloy hand control clamps to the lower part of the steering column and to the pedals. It mounts on the left or right side of the steering column, but will not interfere with the normal operation of the vehicle. A horn and dimmer switch is also located on the handle. To operate, the user pushes the handle forward for brakes or clutch. The device will operate in extreme temperatures, and will fit vehicles with automatic transmissions and foreign models with the steering wheel on the left.

Rehabilitation Equipment and Supply, 4804 North Sheridan Road, Peoria, IL 61614-5928; (309) 676-6054

WHEELCHAIR-ACCESSIBLE MOTOR HOME: Wheelchair-accessible recreational vehicle. Has 30-inch minimum width in all areas; extra-wide door and lift; large bathroom for use from a wheelchair; accessible kitchen with roll-under counter, two-burner stove and sofa beds. Cab area is fully upholstered with reclining captains seats and optional hand controls with six-way powered seat. Outside utilities are accessible from wheelchair.

Wells-Engberg Company, Incorporated, Post Office Box 6388, Rockford, IL 61125-1388; (815) 874-5882 or (800) 642-3628

WELLS ENGBERG DRIVING CONTROL: This device is a hand control for automobiles designed for use by people with disabilities. The brake is operated by pressing the arm of the hand control toward the firewall in a direction parallel to the steering column; The accelerator operates by twisting the grip on the hand control in a counter-clockwise direction. The brake and accelerator can be operated simultaneously for steep grades. The control may be used on any vehicle with an automatic transmission, power steering, and power brakes. The unit is equipped for either left- or right-handed operation and does not affect normal operation of the vehicle. The control mounts on the steering column, brake, and accelerator.

Wright Way, Incorporated, 175 East I-30, Garland, TX 75043; (214) 240-8839

> WRIGHT WAY CONTROL: Chrome-plated hand control operates by pushing toward floor parallel to steering column for brake and by pulling at right angle toward lap for accelerator. Bike-handle grip can be added for better grip. Toggle switches can be attached to hand control for dimmer switch and horn. Hand control bolts to floor and under dash. Conventional cruise control can be attached to this hand control. Switch for cruise control can be adapted to individual driver's needs. Brake and throttle can be applied simultaneously by moving hand control forward and down at the same time. This unit is VA approved.

CLOTHING

Adaptogs, Post Office Box 339, 123 North Washington, Otis, CO 80743; (800) 535-8247 or (303) 246-3761

> CAPE: The Cape, model 148, is waist length with ribbing at the neck designed for women. It has a full-front opening with a Velcro closure. The cape is made of sweatshirt knit fabric cut to drape around the shoulders and provide warmth. Sizes: small, medium, large, extra large, or extra extra large. Colors: prints or solids.

> MEN'S COVER-UP: Men's cover-ups are boxer-style undershorts that may be used as a single garment, or to cover up disposable undergarments. The shorts have full side openings that lay flat for easy dressing. Available with either snap or Velcro closure on both sides. Sizes: small, medium, large, extra large, and extra extra large.

American Health Care Apparel Limited, (800) 252-0584

Avenues Unlimited, 1199 K Avenida Acaso, Camarillo, CA 93012; (800) 848-2837

Buck and Buck, 4115 SW Arroyo Dive, Seattle, WA 98146; (800) 458-0600

Claypool Classics, 586 N. Bank Lane, Lake Forest, IL 60045; (708) 234-4118

TWO-PIECE SUIT: The two-piece suit consists of a man's vest and pants and is designed for easy dressing. The suit is available in corduroy, polyester/cotton, pincord, and twill. The pants feature a drop front with Velcro closure. The vest features Velcro closing under a button front, an opening at one shoulder is optional. Comes in small, medium, large, extra large. Colors: blue or tan.

MEN'S NIGHTSHIRT: This men's nightshirt is tailored with traditional shirtmaker details. Features include: long sleeves with cuffs, below-the-knees length, and ties at the back, or an optional closed back. The nightshirt is made of polyester/cotton. Comes in sizes small (36–38), medium (40–42), large (44–46), or extra large (48–50). Colors: blue stripes, brown tattersall, or red plaid.

Clothes You-Nique Incorporated, Post Office Box 8306, Stockton, CA 95208; (800) 767-7711 or (209) 463-3376

JCPenney Company, Easy Dressing Line, Milwaukee, WI 53263; (800) 222-6161

Promote Real Independence for the Disabled, 391 Long Hill Road, Groton, CT 06340; (203) 445-1448

Rolling Thunder, 1128 Nuuany Avenue, Honolulu, HI 96817; (800) 367-3633

Wardrobe Wagon, Incorporated, 555 Valley Road, Post Office Box 714, West Orange, NJ 07051; (800) WWCARES

Wings, 2239 East 55th Street, Cleveland, OH 44103; (800) 227-6625

DAILY LIVING AIDS

Activeaid Incorporated, One Activaid Road, Post Office Box 359, Redwood Falls, MN 56283-0359; (507) 644-2951 or (800) 533-5330

BEDSIDE COMMODE: The bedside commode is an adjustable-height commode with a removable padded back, full-length arms, rubber-tipped legs, and interchangeable padded seat and commode seat. A closed-front seat or open-ended seat, padded armrests, and a bedpan holder are available. The unit folds when the commode pan is removed. The commode has a chrome-plated finish. Seat height ranges from 21 to 24 inches, seat width is $17^{1}/_{2}$ inches; overall width is $20^{3}/_{16}$ inches. Medicare covered with qualifications.

Adaptability, Post Office Box 515, Colchester, CT 06415-0515; (203) 537-3451 or (800) 243-9232

HANDY HAIRBRUSH: The Handy Hairbrush is a hairbrush with an extended handle and nylon-reinforced natural bristles. The handle has two articulating joints which can be adjusted to a number of positions. The brush extends out to $17^{1}/_{2}$ inches.

Aegis Medical, Incorporated, 10488 West Centennial Road, Littleton, CO 80127; (800) 232-9919

Air Lift Unlimited Incorporated, 1212 Kerr Gulch, Evergreen, CO 80439; (303) 526-0132

Alternate Stoneware, Post Office Box 2071, Charleston, WV 25327-2071; (304) 346-4440

Aqua-Aire International, 2420 Carson Street, Suite 100, Torrance, CA 90501; (213) 320-9379 (collect in California) or (800) 262-6201

Aqua-Tec, Post Office Box 7066, Pittsburgh, PA 15212; (412) 322-7800

Arjo, 6380 West Oakton Street, Morton Grove, IL 60053; (708) 967-0360 or (800) 323-1245

Bath-O-Matic, (800) 423-7886 or (312) 634-2626 (call collect in Illinois)

Bruce Medical Supply, 411 Wavely Oaks Road, Post Office Box 9166, Waltham, MA 02254; (800) 225-8446

Capability Collection, Ways and Means Catalog, 28001 Citron Drive, Romulus, MI 48174; (800) 654-2345

Care Catalog Services, 1877 NE Seventh Street, Portland, OR 97212; (800) 443-7091

Cleo, Incorporated, 3957 Mayfield Road, Cleveland, OH 44121; (216) 382-9700 or (800) 321-0595

Convaid Products, Incorporated, Post Office Box 2458, Palo Verde, CA 90274; (213) 539-6814 (in California) or (800) 552-1020

Duraline, 7 to 13 East Main, Post Office Box 67, Lepsic, OH 45856 (800) 654-3376

Electric Mobility Corporation, 1 Mobility Plaza, Sewell, NJ 08080, (609) 468-0270 or (800) 662-4548

> RELAX 'N' LIFT RECLINER CHAIR: The Relax 'N' Lift Recliner Chair is a recliner chair and seat lift chair designed for use by people who have physical disabilities or who have difficulty seating themselves in or rising from a chair. This motorized recliner tilts forward to ease the user into and out of the chair, keeping the user's arms and back supported. Both standard and deluxe models have hardwood frames, sagless springs, steel lift mechanisms, cord-mounted hand controls, soil-resistant fabric, high reclining back, extended footrest, and a magazine pocket. The deluxe model also includes a heat and vibration massage system.

Everest and Jennings, Incorporated, 1100 Corporate Square Drive, St. Louis, MO 63132-2908; (314) 569-3515 or (800) 235-4661

> FIXED HEIGHT COMMODE WITH REMOVABLE ARMS: Commode chair with full-length swing-out arms, five-inch casters, locks on front casters. Unit has closed-front seat, commode pan, upholstered seat cover and backrest. Medicare covered with qualifications.

Extensions for Independence, 555 Saturn Boulevard, B-368, San Diego, CA 92154; (619) 423-7709

Farberware, 1500 Bassett Avenue, Bronx, NY 10461; (212) 863-8000

> ELECTRIC SKILLET AND GRIDDLE: Stainless-steel fry pan or cast-aluminum griddle, several sizes available. All units have detectable controls and two heat-resistant handles. Completely immersible for cleaning. Stainless-steel electric woks are also available. All units have 120-volt AC.

Fred Sammons Incorporated, A Bissell Healthcare Company, Post Office Box 32, Brookfield, IL 60513-0032

> HIGH SIDE DISH: $7^3/_4$-inch-diameter dish with $1^3/_4$-inch-height vertical wall around half of diameter. Wall slopes to $^1/_2$ inch. Dishwasher-safe. Melamine plastic.

TROUSER PULL: The Quad Quip Trouser Pull is a trouser aid designed to assist individuals pull up pants without bending over. The device consists of plastic hooks for the belt loops and has a series of webbing loops to pull trousers up.

Gladys E. Loeb Foundation, Incorporated, 2002 Forest Hill Drive, Silver Spring, MD 20903; (301) 434-7748

GUARD RAIL RINGS: The Guard Rail Rings are burner guards designed to prevent pots and pans from sliding off range burners. The rings slip into place around the burners. For use on electric range burners only. Two sizes are available to fit burners with diameters of $6^{1}/_{4}$ and $8^{1}/_{8}$ inches.

Guardian Product Incorporated, Division of Sunrise Medical Company, 12800 Wentworth Street, Arleta, CA 91331-4522; (818) 504-2820 or (800) 255-5022

WHEELCHAIR COMMODE: This wheelchair commode comes with a fully padded back and seat with water-repellent vinyl, removable rear wheels, folding back for portability, lightweight aluminum construction, commode pan, push handles, removable armrests, multiple-position commode opening, swing-away removable footrests, five-inch rubber front casters. Available with five-inch rear casters and jack brakes, 24-inch mag or steel-spoke rear wheels, aluminum or plastic-coated hand rims.

Handi Aid Company, Murrieta, CA 92362-8908; (714) 698-0526

VACUUM FEEDING CUP: This vacuum feeding cup permits the individual to control the flow of liquid intake without help or raising his or her head. Finger pressure on the button releases a small amount of fluid and permits controlled feeding. Fluid will not spill if cup tilts. Three sizes available: 4, 6, and 8 ounces.

Home Delivery Incontinent Supplies Company, Post Office Box 52039, St. Louis, MO 63136; (314) 389-4134 (Missouri or Canada) or (800) 538-1036

Independent Living Aids, Incorporated, 11 Commercial Court, Plainview, NY 11803; (800) 262-7827

Lumex Incorporated, 100 Spence Street, Bay Shore, NY 11706-2290; (516) 273-2200 or (800) 645-5272

CUTLERY SET: This cutlery set is designed for persons with diminished hand strength and range of motion. Lightweight utensils with broad plastic handles; knife is at right angle to handle and folds; fork is 7.8 inches; and spoon is 8.9 inches.

HANDY EXTENDERS: Long-handled bath and grooming utensils. Handle has two joints which adjust to any angle. Folds for storage. Oval profile with longitudinal grooves for easy grip. Nylon with plastic handle. Utensils include comb, hairbrush, bathbrush, extra-long bathbrush, nail file, and washcloth.

Maddak Incorporated, Six Industrial Road, Pequannock, NJ 07440; (201) 628-7600 or (800) 443-4926

DENTAL FLOSS HOLDER: The Floss Aid Dental Floss Holder is a Y-shaped frame designed to allow persons with arthritis, limitations of manual dexterity, or the use of only one hand to floss their own teeth effectively. The handle measures six inches long.

SCOOP DISH: The Melamine Scooper Dish is a bowl dish designed for persons with limited muscle control or the use of only one hand. These dishes have contoured lips to help in scooping food onto utensils. The oval-shaped dishes are dishwasher safe, made of break-resistant plastic, and feature brown decorator patterns. The dishes are available with self-adhesive, nonslip neoprene foam. The dishes come in three sizes: bowl ($5\,^1/_2$ by $6\,^1/_2$ inches by $2\,^3/_4$ inches deep on high end); medium-sized dish (6 by $7\,^1/_2$ inches by $1\,^3/_4$ inches deep on high end), and dinner-sized dish (8 by 10 inches by $1\,^7/_8$ inches deep on the high end).

SELF-LEVELING SWIVEL UTENSILS: The self-leveling swivel utensils are designed so that the eating implement always remains upright when placed into the mouth, even if the hand is raised at a steep angle. The utensils are made of stainless steel mounted by a swivel pin to a built-up handle. Double stops prevent excessive swing. A fork, teaspoon, and soup spoon are available, and are all dishwasher safe.

SELECT SPECIAL KITCHEN UTENSILS: The select special utensils are a collection of cutlery designed for individuals who do not have full use of their arms and hands. The eight pieces are made of highly polished, heavy-duty stainless steel with dishwasher-safe handles. Knife edges are serrated and curved, forks have four tines, and spoons are relatively deep.

ZIPPER AID: The Zipper Aid is a long-handled zipper pull designed to assist individuals with back-closing zippers. The wooden stick has a plastic handle and a Z-shaped hook for catching zipper pull tabs. Twenty small rings are supplied for attaching to zipper tabs. Stick is 20 inches long.

Medical Line Warehouse, 6130 Clark Center Avenue #103, Saratoga, FL 34238; (813) 924-2058 or (800) 247-2256

ROCKER KNIFE AND FORK: The Rocker Knife and Fork is a combination knife and fork designed to simplify cutting and eating for individuals with the use of only one hand. The knife has a curved blade. The fork has three tines. Each are made of stainless steel with solid handles.

Power Access Corporation, Bridge Street Post Office Box 235, Collinsville, CT 06022; (800) 344-0088

Sanlex International Incorporated, Post Office Box 14717, Dayton, OH 45414; (800) 424-1224

Ways and Means, 28001 Citron Drive, Romulus, MI 48174; (800) 654-2345

William's Connection International, Post Office Box 3508, San Clemente, CA 92672; (714) 244-2617

COMMUNICATION AIDS/
COMMUNICATION BOARDS

ACS Communications, 250 Technology Circle, Scotts Valley, CA 95066; (800) 538-0742

Ameriphone, 1140-F North Kraemer Boulevard, Anaheim, CA 92806; (714) 632-5028

AT&T Conversant Systems, 6200 East Broad Street, Columbus, OH 43212; (800) 233-1222

AT&T National Special Needs Center (AT&T NSNC), 2001 Route 46, Suite 310, Parsippany, NJ 07054-1315; (800) 233-1222

AT&T, 295 North Maple Avenue, Basking Ridge, NJ 07920; (800) 233-1222 (for hearing-assist)

Baggeboda Press, 107 North Pine Street, Little Rock, AR 72205; (501) 664-8183

Buchart-Horn, Incorporated, 55 South Richland Avenue, Post Office Box M-55, York, PA 17405; (717) 843-5561

Cleo, Incorporated, 3957 Mayfield Road, Cleveland, OH 44121; (216) 382-9700 or (800) 321-0595

Command Telephone System, 5600 N. Antioch Road, Kansas City, MO 64119; (816) 453-2010

Communication Skill Builders, 383 East Bellevue, Post Office Box 42050, Tucson, AZ 85733; (602) 323-7500

PRODUCTS AVAILABLE: Sign-language coloring books, self-talk communication boards, sign-language training, self-talk stickers.

Crestwood Company, 6625 North Sydney Place, Milwaukee, WI 53209-3259; (414) 352-5678

SCREAMER ALARM: The screamer alarm is a switch-activated call signal that alerts family members or professional staff to an individual's immediate need for help. The high-pitched pulsing sound is far reaching. The alarm comes with a 10-foot cord so it can be placed in a hallway if needed for the sound to reach even greater distances. Powered by a 9-volt battery. Switch not included.

VOICE-INPUT CONTROL SWITCH: The voice switch is a voice- or sound-input control switch that will turn various devices on and off. The switch has a sensitivity control range and two selectors. Monitoring, requires continuous talking to operate the switch, and the user must stop talking to shut the switch off. This selector may also be used for breath control; the first sound turns the switch on, the second sound turns it off. This switch can be used with communication devices, toys, or other devices that use control switches.

DQP, Incorporated, 14167 Meadow Drive, Grass Valley, CA 95945; (916) 477-1234

Eagle Marketing, 5321 South Sheridan #15, Tulsa, OK 74145; (918) 663-4477

> BOOK HOLDER: Plastic book holder/copy holder, easel back, adjusts to any angle and folds flat, foam grippers on top and bottom hold document open yet allow pages to turn easily. Adjustable T-bar accommodates any publication higher than $7^1/_4$ inches. Holds copy, magazines, softback and hardback books. Includes extenders for thicker and smaller publications.

F. Keep Company, 22501 Mount Eden Road, Saratoga, CA 95070; (408) 248-2579 or (408) 741-5368

Fred Sammons, Incorporated, 2915 Walkent NW, Department 636, Grand Rapids, MI 49504; (616) 784-0208 (for hearing-assist)

Fred Sammons, Incorporated, 145 Tower Drive, Burr Ridge, IL 60521; (800) 323-7305 (for communications devices)

Fred Sammons, Incorporated, Box 32, Brookfield, IL 60513-0032; (800) 323-5547 (for reading aids)

> BOOK MAID: The Book Maid is an adjustable-angle book holder designed to be used in a sitting or lying position. The device consists of a lightweight aluminum frame with a Plexiglas tray. The tray is 8 by 12 inches with a $1^1/_2$-inch lip.

Garid, Incorporated, 10180 Viking Drive, Eden Prairie, MN 55344; (612) 941-5464

Help Me Help Myself Communication Aids, 342 Acre Avenue, Brownsburg, IN 46112; (317) 852-4427

Imaginart Communication Products, 25680 Oakwood Street, Post Office Box 1868, Idlewild, CA 92349; (714) 659-5905

Innocomp Innovative Computer Applications, 33195 Wagon Wheel, Solon, OH 44139; (216) 248-6206

Mayer-Johnson Company, Post Office Box 1579, Solana Beach, CA 92075; (619) 481-2489

Pitts Corporation, 4620 North 650, East Provo, UT 84604;
(801) 225-6441

EYEGAZE COMMUNICATOR: Eye-Com is a portable non-electronic communication aid. The operator of the device stands near the user and gazes at the user through the center of the device. The operator rotates the letter wheel until the pointer rests on the desired letter. The user then gives a signal (such as an eye blink) to signal the operator to stop. Letters are then recorded on paper by the operator, and the process is repeated until an entire word or thought is expressed. Both right-handed and left-handed models of Eye-Com are available. The device measures 16 by 16 inches and weighs one pound.

Pleasure Endeavors, 375 Laguna Honda Boulevard, Room 323, San Francisco, CA 94116; (415) 759-2320

R. D. Clark, Incorporated, Box 22, Bowling Green, IN 47833;
(812) 986-2178

Radio Shack, Fort Worth, TX 76102 (contact your local dealer)

Sparr Telephone Arm Company, Post Office Box 143, Allamuchy, NJ 07820; (904) 423-5971

TASH (The Association for Persons with Severe Handicaps) 7010 Roosevelt Way NE, Seattle, WA 98115; (206) 523-8446

Tiger Communications System, Incorporated, 115 East Broad Street #325, Rochester, NY 14604; (716) 454-5134

Typewriting Institute for the Handicapped, 3102 W. Augusta Avenue, Phoenix, AZ 85051; (602) 939-5344

Variety Ability Systems, Incorporated (VASI), 3701 Danforth Avenue, Scarbourough, Toronto, Ontario MIN 2G2 Canada; (416) 698-1415

CRUTCHES, CANES, AND WALKERS

Advantage, 22633 Ellinwood Drive, Torrance, CA 90505;
(213) 540-8197 (voice)

George E. Alexander and Son, Incorporated, 45 Lower Main Street, Sunapee, NH 03782; (603) 763-2221

AUXILIARY CRUTCH: Adjustable, wooden crutch, laminated or solid. Sizes: extra-long adult, adult, medium adult, youth, child, baby. Medicare covered with qualifications.

Bruce Medical Supply, 411 Waverly Oaks Road, Post Office Box 9166, Waltham, MA 02254; (800) 225-8446

Cleo, Incorporated, 3857 Mayfield Road, Cleveland, OH 44121; (216) 382-9700 or (800) 321-0595

WALKER WITH PLATFORM ARM SUPPORT: Adjustable four-legged frame with low cross brace. Has vinyl-covered, foam-padded wooden platforms with vertical handles for forearm use. Base area $22^{1}/_{2}$ by $16^{1}/_{2}$ inches. Adjustable height 33 to 37 inches. Medicare covered with qualifications.

Conkle and Conkle Manufacturing, 212 Walnut Street, Harrod, OH 45850; (419) 648-3328

NIGHT LIGHT FOR WALKING DEVICES: The Night Light for Walking Devices is a light for canes, walkers, crutches or wheelchairs. The unit has a flat back and may be attached to equipment with Velcro. It has a long throw toggle switch for activation. This item produces a spot of light for illuminating the surrounding area. It is powered by 2 AA batteries, with 2.4-volt bulb. The weight is $5^{1}/_{2}$ ounces with batteries.

DMA USA, Incorporated, 306A Dallas Drive, Denton, TX 76201; (817) 383-8393 or (800) 362-8722

ADJUSTABLE WALKER: Walkers with aluminum frames. Adjustable height 33 to 36 inches with two front wheels, width $26^{3}/_{8}$ inches, depth $15^{3}/_{4}$ inches. Plastic handgrips, rubber tips on legs.

Fred Sammons, Incorporated, 2915 Walkent NW, Department 636, Grand Rapids, MI 49504; (616) 784-0208

Guardian Products, Incorporated, 12800 Wentworth Street, Arleta, CA 91331-4522; (818) 504-2820 or (800) 255-5022

GUIDE-LINE SAFE T CRUTCH: Height adjustable aluminum crutch with molded plastic armrest and adjustable plastic handgrip.

Adult size 46 to 60 inches. Youth 38 to 47 inches. Child 29 to 38 inches.

Maddak Incorporated, 6 Industrial Road, Pequannock, NJ 07440; (201) 628-7600 or (800) 443-4926

CANE HOLDER: The Cane Clip with table clamp is a cane holder designed to accommodate any size cane securely, while allowing easy release. The device has a spring-action clamp with grooved, soft plastic rollers that will not mar the cane's shaft. The rubber-lined clamp fits onto table tops or counters up to $1^3/4$ inches thick and is secured by a clamping screw with a swivel guide. Dimensions: $3^3/4$ by $3^1/2$ by 2 inches.

Preco Products, 8019 Flood Road, Baltimore, MD 21222; (301) 285-1135 or (800) 426-6503

UNDERARM CRUTCH: Anodized aluminum auxiliary crutch. Adjustable handgrip, four positions. Adjustable height, wing nuts. Anodized finish. Adult sizes 42 to 60 inches; youth, 29 to 41 inches.

Maneuverability, 4015 Avenue U (Coleman Street), Brooklyn, NY 11234; (718) 692-0909

Tubular Fabricators Industry, Incorporated, 600 West Wythe Street, Petersburg, VA 23803; (800) 526-0178

FOLDING SEAT WALKER: Four-legged folding adjustable walker with folding seat. The walker has 4-inch wheels on front legs. Automatic snap clip holds heavily padded vinyl-covered seat in up position. Height of walker adjusts from 32 to 36 inches. Walker is 23 inches wide. Depth is 19 inches open and $8^1/2$ inches folded. Weight: 9 pounds.

Winnie Walker Company, 505 North del Prado Boulevard, Cape Coral, FL 33909-2244; (813) 772-5155 or (800) 544-5155

ADJUSTABLE WHEELED WALKER WITH FOLDING SEAT: This is an adjustable wheel walker designed for use by people with mobility impairments. This four-wheeled walker features large wheels for easy handling, one-touch locking handbrakes, and a padded seat. An optional carrying basket and tray are available. Dimensions are $27^1/2$ by $22^1/2$ inches, the height adjusts from 31 to

41 inches. The seat is 6¹/₂ inches deep and 14 inches wide. Weight: 20 pounds.

Electric Scooters

Alpha Mobility Incorporated, 4265 Kellway Circle, Dallas, TX 75244-2033; (214) 407-8400 or (800) 749-5444

ALPHA TRI KART: Three-wheeled electric-powered cart used primarily indoors. Front-wheel drive, 12-volt system uses gel cell battery, removable arms, 360-degree swivel seat with lock, 6-amp battery charger. Speed is 3 mph, forward and reverse. Parking brake lever for rear wheels. T steering column can be locked into drive head. Lever drive control on handle of steering tiller can be used with one hand. Overall length is 36 inches, width 18 inches. Weight without battery, seat, or steering column is 33 pounds; total weight 68 pounds. Aluminum and stainless-steel construction. Solid rubber tires, front plastic bumper. Options include wider arms, lower arms, crutch holders, 3-inch longer base; 24-volt model available. Medicare covered with qualifications. (Specify powered wheelchair.)

Amigo Mobility International Incorporated, 6693 Dixie Highway, Bridgeport, MI 48722; (517) 777-0910 or (800) 821-2710

AMIGO FWD SCOOTER: The Amigo FWD is a three-wheeled powered wheelchair alternative, designed for indoor and outdoor use. The frame is painted steel platform with a wheel base of 31 inches. Overall length is 37 inches and the width is 24 inches with dual rear wheels. It is operated by a lever control in an oval-shaped handlebar on a telescoping double-adjustable handle. It is front-wheel drive (FWD). The padded seat is height adjustable, swivels 360 degrees, and locks in any position. The seat is removable without tools. A power seat lift is available as an option, as well as a reclining back and tilting seat. The brakes are dynamic and regenerative with choice of right- or left-side brake lock. The wheels are dual 6-inch flat-free rear wheels and 6-inch flat-free front tires. It is powered by a 12-volt electrical system using one battery including a battery charger. Maximum speed is 3.4 miles per hour for a maximum range of 16 miles. Variable speed, forward and reverse.

Dignified Corporation, Post Office Box 337, Mantu, NJ 08051; (800) 548-7905

Electric Mobility, 1 Mobility Plaza, Sewell, NJ 08080; (609) 468-0270 or (800) 662-4548

HEAVY DUTY RASCAL SCOOTER: The Heavy Duty Rascal Scooter is a three-wheeled scooter designed for use by people who have lower-extremity disabilities or limited mobility. These scooters have all-terrain capability and come standard with a removable front basket, a carryall rear basket, voltmeter/fuel gauge, removable adjustable swivel handlebars, on/off switch, and electric push-button horn. The unit is 44 inches long by 25 inches wide and has a 29.5-inch wheel base. The unit breaks down into three easily handled sub-sections for ease of transport. It has a speed of 4.5 miles per hour with a maximum range of 20 miles and a climbing capacity of 25 percent (14 degrees). Weight: 141.5 pounds with batteries. Comments: This product may be covered by medical insurance or Medicare if purchaser qualifies.

Fortress, 3750 Chesswood Drive, Downsview, Ontario M3J2W6 Canada; (800) 263-1408

Hugh Macmillan Rehabilitation Centre, 350 Rumsey Road, Toronto, Ontario M4G 1R8 Canada; (416) 425-6220 or (800) 363-2440

MINIATURE POWERED VEHICLE: Three-wheeled child's powered cart, eight-position joystick controller steering tiller. Two 12-volt motors, two 6-volt, 2-amp hour acid batteries, estimated operational time 7 hours per charge. Two 10-inch pneumatic drive wheels in rear; front wheel 4-inch solid caster. Two speeds, low approximately 1.6 km per hour; high approximately 3.2 km per hour. Overall length 36 inches, width 21 inches. Seat and back are vinyl upholstered with two safety belts. The seat system is detach-able for installation of other postural supports. Seat reclines 20 degrees and has 3-inch adjustable height for growth. Rear wheels de-clutch for free-wheeling; push handles included. Developed for children two to five years old with disabilities such as Mus-cular Dystrophy, Spinal Muscular Atrophy, Spina Bifida, and Cerebral Palsy.

Invacare Corporation, 899 Cleveland Street, Elyria, OH 44036-2125; (216) 329-6237

Jubilee Scooter Incorporated, 324 Lake Side Drive, Suite A, Foster City, CA 94404; (415) 571-5323

Mobility Engineering, 5555 South Country Club Road, Tucson, AZ 85706; (502) 889-8636 or (800) 767-2668

THE BOBCAT SCOOTER: The Bobcat is a powered wheelchair alternative. This three-wheeled scooter disassembles for transport and storage. The frame is steel with overall dimensions of 44 inches long, $23^1/_2$ inches wide with a 33-inch turning radius. The scooter has an adjustable tiller with an easy-release lever. The seat is an uncontoured cushion seat and flip down back. Armrests are padded desk style. The brakes are automatic electric parking brake. It is powered with standard U-1–size gel cell batteries with speeds up to $5^1/_2$ mph and a range of 10 to 20 miles on one charge. Weight 143 pounds with batteries. The heaviest part when disassembled is 38 pounds.

Motion Power, 2842 Business Park Avenue, Fresno, CA 93727; (209) 292-2171

Okoboji Industries, Rural Route 3, Box 125, Milford, IA 51351; (800) 841-2222

Ortho-Kinetics, Incorporated, Post Office Box 1647, Waukesha, WI 53187; (800) 558-7786, ext. 381

Palmer Industries, Post Office Box CN 707, Endicott, NY 13760; (607) 754-1954 or (800) 847-1304

C F Struck Corporation, W51 North 545 Struck Lane, Box 307, Cedarburg, WI 53012; (414) 377-3300

MINI BEEP SCOOTER: Powered wheelchair alternative designed primarily for indoor use or outdoor use on hard, level surfaces. High-performance option adds stability and power for outdoor use on more rugged terrain. Can climb slopes of 5 degrees. Mini Beep has three 8-inch wheels, front-wheel drive for maneuverability, two speeds in forward and reverse (1 mph and 3.5 mph). Machine operates by throttle button and has squeeze brake handgrip and brake lock. Seat rotates 360 degrees with lock positions every 90 degrees. Seat height adjusts 6 inches up and 1 inch down, adjusts 3 inches front to rear to allow extra leg room. Steering handles constructed of two columns, for support when transferring. Options include throttle control on left or right, brake on left or right, gel battery, high performance package. The unit is 34 inches high and 20 inches wide, with a wheel base of $30^3/_4$ inches, and an overall length of 41 inches.

Supercruiser, Incorporated, 23870 Pine Street #1, Newhall, CA 91321-3111; (805) 255-6635

> FOOT-PROPELLED CART: Foot-powered scooter has four large wheels, a wide foot platform, a stable handle, and powerful brakes. Handle folds down for easy storage. Comes fully assembled. Very easy to ride. Develops strength, coordination, and self-esteem.

Vessa Limited, 1103 Musser Street, Muscatine, IA 52761; (800) 728-6624

Voyager, 527 West Colfax, South Bend, IN 46601; (219) 288-0511

ENVIRONMENTAL CONTROL SYSTEMS/DEVICES

CyberLYNX Computer Products, Incorporated, 4828 Sterling Drive, Boulder, CO 80301; (303) 444-7733

Dimango Products, 7258 Kensington Road, Brighton, MI 48116; (313) 486-0770

> OFF/ON REMOTE SWITCH: Off/On Remote Switch is a system consisting of a small hand-held transmitter unit with a button on top and a receiver unit that plugs into a wall outlet. The appliance to be controlled is plugged into the receiver, and the user can turn it on and off at a distance of up to 50 feet by pressing the button on the transmitter unit. Three different frequencies of receivers with corresponding transmitters are available: a lamp model, an appliance model, and a motor and fan model.

EKEG Electronics Company, Limited, Post Office Box 46199, Station G, Vancouver, British Columbia, V6R 4G5 Canada; (604) 685-7817

Fortress Scientific, 61 Miami Street, Buffalo, NY 14204; (800) 263-1408

LC Technologies, Incorporated, 4415 Glenn Rose Street, Fairfax, VA 22032; (703) 425-7509

Mastervoice, 10523 Humbolt Street, Los Alamitos, CA 90720; (310) 594-6581 or (800) 628-5837

> BUTLER-IN-A-BOX: A voice-activated environmental control system with speech output that allows users hands-free operation

of appliances, lights, and telephone. Once the user has trained the Butler to recognize particular utterances, these utterances can be used as commands to activate various appliances: lights, TV, stereo, electric beds, and the like. Timers (included) can also be set to turn appliances on or off at particular times. Appliances are activated remotely using X-10 remote-control modules. A telephone is built in, allowing the user to remotely dial, answer, and use the system as a speaker phone. Butler-In-a-Box can also be programmed to detect the presence of intruders and request that they identify themselves. Options: extras include a voice mouse (for retrieving data from an IBM computer), and ICI infrared controller interface, the RAM pack, the voice cartridge, and the controller. For use with IBM PC computers.

Prentke Romich Company, 1022 Heyl Road, Wooster, OH 44691; (216) 262-1984 or (800) 642-8255

Quartet Technology, Incorporated, 52 Davis Road, Tyngsboro, MA 01879; (508) 692-9313

ENVIRONMENTAL CONTROL UNIT: Simplicity Series 5 is a voice-input-controlled environmental power unit that can be used to operate lights, appliances, phones, electric beds, television, VCR, cable box, and accessories (page turners, door openers, etc.). The user selects appliances and control functions through voice command, and can also train and retrain the system through voice-control alone. Additional lamp and appliance modules may be added to the basic unit. The equipment works through standard house wiring, and operates up to an hour on battery backup in case of power failure.

Safko International, Incorporated, Lon S. Safko, Route 4, Box 4028-A, Kennewick, WA 99337; (509) 627-0745

TASH, Incorporated (Technical Aids and Systems for the Handicapped), 70 Gibson Drive, Unit 1, Markham, Ontario L3R 2Z3 Canada; (416) 475-2212

X-10 (USA), Incorporated, 185A LeGrand Avenue, Northvale, NJ 07647; (201) 784-9700

Home Modifications

American National Standards Institute, 1430 Broadway, New York, NY 10018; (212) 642-4990 (ask for Pamphlet No. A117.1)

Arjo Century Incorporated, 8130 Lehieg Avenue, Morton Grove, IL 60053; (708) 967-0360 or (800) 323-1245

> HYDRAULIC TRANSFER LIFT RIDE CHAIR: Person can be placed on seat while lying in bed, brought to a sitting position and safety arm and backrest lowered around person. Some assistance from the person is required. Lift is hydraulically adjustable, low base with casters. Seat can be lowered into elevating bathtub or used as a commode seat for toilet. Bed and holder attached. Stretcher can be attached to lift in place of seat. Person being transported must have fairly good trunk stability.

Barrier Free Environments, Post Office Box 30634, Raleigh, NC 27622; (919) 782-7823

Bathing Aids to the Handicapped, 10-C Escondido Village, Escondido Road, Stanford, CA 94305; (415) 857-1053

Bow Enterprises, Incorporated, 25 East Main Street, Santa Barbara, CA 93101; (805) 966-6799

Braun Corporation, 1014 South Monticello, Post Office Box 310, Winamac, IN 46996; (219) 946-6157 or (800) 843-5438

> ROLL IN SHOWER: Fiberglass shower stall $4^1/_2$ feet square; entry ramp and exit lip for water retention. Molded shelf. Installed in four pieces: base and three wall panels. Single lever water controls hand shower. Options: barrier-free shower door, safety-mix shower head, wall-mounted shower seat, grab bars.

Comfortably Yours, 61 West Hunter Avenue, Maywood, NJ 07607; (201) 368-0400

Eastern Paralyzed Veterans Association, 75-20 Astoria Boulevard, Jackson Heights, NY 11370-1178; (718) 803-EPVA

Econol Stairway Lift Corporation, 2513 Center Street, Cedar Falls, IA 50613; (319) 277-4777

Flinchbough Company, 390 Eberts Lane, York, PA 17403;
(717) 854-7720

G. E. Miller Incorporated, 54 Nepperhan Avenue, Yonkers, NY 10701;
(914) 969-4036 or (800) 431-2924

SHOWER STOOL: Low stool with large suction tips on legs.
Waterproof, plywood seat, round edges. No back support.

Garaventa Limited, Post Office Box L-1, Blaine, WA 98230;
(604) 594-0422 or (800) 663-6556

STAIR-TRAC: The Garaventa Stair-trac is a portable wheelchair
stair lift designed for interior or outdoor use to allow an attendant to
easily move a wheelchair user up and down most stair surfaces. The
device fits most crossbrace wheelchairs, and will adapt to a child's
narrow wheelchair. The device consists of a folding L-shaped unit
with steel-belted caterpillar tracks on the bottom side to securely
grip stairs, auxiliary wheels for flat surface travel, and a handle
with the control mechanisms on the upright side. The wheelchair
is backed over the tracks and handle-lifted upright. The handle is
attached to the wheelchair with clamps. Ascending or descending
the stairs is initiated with a push button that engages a high-
reduction gear drive 12-volt battery-powered motor. A gel cell
battery charger is included for the two 6-volt batteries. Maximum
stair slope is 35 degrees at a speed of 21 feet going up stairs and 25
feet per minute going down stairs. The unit is $36\frac{1}{2}$ by 58 by 25
inches, with a weight of 119 pounds. Options include a ramp for
loading into and out of the car trunk.

Ted Hoyer and Company, 2222 Minnesota Street, Oshkosh, WI 54901;
(414) 231-7970

HOYER BATHLIFT: Jack-type hydraulic lift device, user or
attendant operated, clamps on edge of bathtub. Commode-type seat,
or fiberglass bucket seat. No armrests. Optional floor mount available. Maximum lift capacity is 250 pounds.

Haas and Alber USA Incorporated, Post Office Box 690, Plaistow,
NH 03865; (603) 382-1660 or (800) 222-9181

POWERED STAIR TRANSPORT FOR WHEELCHAIR: The
Scalamobil Wheelchair Stair Climbing System is a powered stair

transport for wheelchairs. It is designed to transport wheelchair users up and down staircases. The unit is compatible with almost all manual wheelchairs. To connect the unit, the wheelchair is backed into the adapter's wheelguards and secured with a clamping system. A padded headrest assures the passenger's comfort. The unit may be used on any completely dry staircase, including those that are carpeted, made of wood, marble, plastic, metal, and the like. The unit will fit on curving staircases or narrow steps depending on the wheelchair size. The unit operates on a 12-volt system with vapor-proof batteries.

International Healthcare Products, 4222 South Pulaski Road, Chicago, IL 60632; (312) 247-7422 or (800) 423-7886

BATH-O-MATIC HYDROCUSHION: The Bath-O-Matic Hydrocushion is a water-inflatable cushion used as a bath lift that connects to the tub faucet or shower head, designed for those who have difficulty standing. The cushion is placed in the tub and filled with warm water. After transferring to the cushion, the valve on the cushion is opened and the cushion deflates, filling the bathtub with water. After bathing, water is drained from the tub and the cushion is refilled with water. The bather is raised to a sitting position. The cushion is constructed of heavy-duty medical-grade vinyl. Included is a tote bag for storage or travel. Backrest with seatbelt available. Holds 25 gallons of water and lifts up to 300 pounds.

Invacare Corporation, Post Office Box 4028, 899 Cleveland Street, Elyria, OH 44036-2125; (216) 329-6000 or (800) 333-6900

PORTABLE PATIENT LIFT: Patient lift with removable mast. Two models of bases available: U or C shaped. Boom has standard angled bar to attach straps or chains of slings. Offset mast centers patient over base and minimizes swaying during elevation. Small hydraulic cylinder with spring-loaded release valve which is in a constantly closed position unless positively engaged. Pump handle can be rotated side to side and is operated vertically. Maximum load 350 pounds. Four 5-inch casters. C base: 26 inches wide, 8 inches high, 40 inches long. U base: $21^3/_4$ to 40 inches wide, 8 inches high, 38 inches long. Boom height $44^1/_2$ to 71 inches high. Boom length $30^3/_4$ inches. Mast height $51^3/_4$ inches.

ITEC, 5482 Business Drive, Unit C, Huntington Beach, CA 92649; (714) 898-9005 or (800) 622-ITEC

J and S Kogen Builders, Incorporated, Joe Kogen, Vice President, Post Office Box 1700, Highland Park, IL 60035; (847) 831-0544

Maddak, Incorporated, 6 Industrial Road, Pequannock, NJ 07440; (201) 628-7600 or (800) 443-4926

> DOOR KNOB OPENER: The Maddahook Door Knob Opener is a handle turner designed to assist individuals with limited hand strength or dexterity to manipulate many kinds of knobs and handles more easily. The opener consists of a semicircular steel bar covered with vinyl mounted on a built-up plastic handle. A strap to go around the back of the hand is also added for security. The handle is 5 inches long by $7/8$ inches in diameter; overall length is $7^3/4$ inches.

Motor Development Corporation, 9340 Buell Street, Downey, CA 90241; (213) 862-6741

> PARALLEL BARS: Adult-folding parallel bars. Chrome-plated handrails on vinyl-coated steel bases. Height adjustable $27^1/2$ to $38^1/2$ inches in 1-inch increments. Overall length 8 feet. Width $31^1/2$ inches, width between upright posts adjusts to maximum of 21 inches. Folds to 8 inches wide for storage. Additional 4-foot sections available.

New York State Office of Vocational Rehabilitation, (800) 222-JOBS or (800) 222-5627

Porto-Lift Corporation, Post Office Box 5, Higgins Lake, MI 48627-0005; (517) 821-6688

Ramsey and Associates, Post Office Box 220, Vilonia, AR 72173; (501) 796-2981

Safe-T-Bath, 184 Millbury Avenue, Millbury, MA 01527; (508) 865-2361

Stannah Stairlifts, 227 South Street, Hopkinton, MA 01748; (800) UPSTAIR, ext. 648

> STANNAH STAIRLIFT: The Stannah Stairlift will fit most types of stairs, whether straight or curved. The stairlift rail sits on the stair and is not attached to the wall and as such there is no need for structural alteration. For further information, call or write directly to the manufacturer.

United Cerebral Palsy, Project Open Door, 1770 Stillwell Avenue, Bronx, NY 10469; (212) 519-5181

HOSPITAL AND ORTHOPEDIC EQUIPMENT FOR THE HOME

American Hospital Supply Corporation, 6600 West Touhy Avenue, Chicago, IL 60648; (804) 424-5200

ALTERNATING AIR PRESSURE MATTRESS: Mattress consists of 40 transverse tubes within a vinyl casing. Air pressure is pumped through them in alternating patterns every 15 seconds. In addition, the system sends a continuous stream of air through perforations in the air tubes and then through a 19-millimeter foam mattress. The power unit has preattached air hoses, 40 inches wide by 80 inches long and fits on top of a standard hospital mattress. Medicare covered with qualifications.

Hard Manufacturing Company Incorporated, 230 Grider Street, Buffalo, NY 14215-3797; (716) 893-1800 or (800) 873-4273

THE MONROE MOTORIZED CRIB/BED: The Monroe Bed is a motorized bed designed for user safety, caregiver accessibility, and compatibility with mist tent respirators, and IV accessories. This bed has cleanable vinyl panels to provide containment while allowing access to the occupant from all four sides. The bed is suitable for home care as well as hospital use. It can achieve all required nursing positions including hyperextension and cardiac care. The electric configuration has a high-low function to allow easy wheelchair transfers and work height adjustments. A user hand control, nurse's lockout and control panel are standard. Available in two sizes. One has a 36 by 68-inch sleeping surface for younger patients; the other has an adult sleeping surface of 36 by 80 inches.

Healthflex Incorporated, 127 Bowen Road, Bennington, VT 05201-2017; (802) 447-2366 or (800) 782-8889

PRESSURE GUARD FOAM AND AIR FLOTATION MATTRESS: Spinal support and pressure-relieving mattress that fits on existing bed frame. A system of inflated air cylinders and wooden slats supports foam that evenly distributes weight and relieves pressure, aiding in the prevention of decubitus ulcers and providing spinal support. King, queen, double, twin, and hospital sizes.

Hill-Rom, A Hillenbrand Industry Company, 4349 Corporate Road, Charleston, SC 29405; (800) 638-2546

ACUCAIR CONTINUOUS AIRFLOW MATTRESS SYSTEM: The ACUCAIR Continuous Airflow System constantly provides pressure reduction over the entire body contact area through a feature called Digital Logic Circuitry. This state-of-the-art electronics automatically adjusts pressure whenever the patient changes position so a constant, predetermined level of pressure is maintained. The mattress system provides solutions to all causes of pressure ulcers: pressure, moisture, shear, and friction. Carefully placed micro air vents allow air to escape to keep the patient dry. The breathable fabric helps reduce shear and friction. The system comes in two basic models—an airflow system which is used with a standard mattress and a complete mattress system. This is covered by Medicare if qualifications are met.

Jefferson Industries Incorporated, 1985 Rutgers University Boulevard, Lakewood, NJ 08701; (908) 905-9001 or (800) 257-5145

STOP LEAK GEL FLOTATION MATTRESS: The Stop Leak Gel Flotation Mattress is a mattress surface overlay designed to reduce the risk of decubitus ulcers. The pad features five internal partitions to eliminate motion and increase stability. The mattress is made of vinyl and nylon material developed to prevent punctures from becoming large holes. A powered gel concentrate and water are put into the mattress and mixed to form the gel. If mattress does puncture, the gel beads up to prevent leakage.

Medi Athleti-K Incorporated, 2175 Place Thimens, Ville St-Laurent, Quebec H4R 1K8 Canada; (514) 331-7214 or (800) 361-6857

THERAPEUTIC PILLOW: The Therapeutic Pillow is a cervical pillow designed to support the head and neck area. The pillow has small cylindrical extensions on opposite sides of the rectangular foam support, and comes with a cover. Dimensions: 56 by 45 centimeters.

Motor Development Corporation, 9340 Buell Street, Downey, CA 90241; (213) 862-6741

AIR MATTRESS: This air flotation mattress has a reinforced vinyl cover that is inflated by a constant flow of air. This constant flow provides equalized exterior surface pressure. Double-zippered vents control pressure. 110-volt blower included.

ADJUSTABLE STANDER: The adjustable stander is a prone board designed to provide support to the user. This product includes three adjustable boards on a main support. The kneeboard and chestboard are padded with carpet with two belts which extend from the boards to provide support. The attached hingeboard fastens to a table using two C'clamps.

Nova Health Systems Incorporated, 409 VPR Commerce Center, Blackwood, NJ 08012; (609) 228-8833 or (800) 225-6682

NOVA AIR FLOTATION SYSTEM: Alternating air pressure flotation mattress surface for prevention of decubitus ulcers. Features airflow to provide skin ventilation; box-fitted end panels for attachment to hospital mattress; feature for uninterrupted airflow while patient is in any position; sleeved air hoses with positive locking system; concentric arc design for massaging action. Alternate sets of cells inflate and deflate twice each minute. Consists of power unit (14 by 9 inches) and Nova mattress (38 by 84 inches). Special needs pad (20 by 36 inches) also available.

Neuropedic, 120 North Abington Road, Clarks Summit, PA 18411; (717) 586-1323

MOTORIZED ADJUSTABLE BED: The Neuropedic Electric Adjustable Bed is a motorized bed frequently used by persons requiring a larger adjustable bed than the standard hospital or twin size. An anti-decubitus Neuropedic mattress is standard. This product comes in twin to king sizes. Side rails are optional. This product is Medicare covered with qualifications.

Smith and Davis Manufacturing Company, 1100 Corporate Square Drive, St. Louis, MO 63132-2908; (314) 569-3515 or (800) 788-3633

MOTORIZED BED: This hospital-style bed has all-electric adjustments, a double cross bar construction for attachment of aids, and a six-button hand-held control. Laminated ends. Mattress size is

36 by 80 inches. Does not include mattress or side rails. Medicare covered with qualifications.

SEMI-ELECTRIC MOTORIZED BED: Same bed as described above except semi-electric (high and low function operated by single crank at foot end).

Southwest Technologies Incorporated, 2018 Baltimore, Kansas City, MO 64108; (816) 221-2442 or (800) 247-9951

ELASTO-GEL LUMBAR PILLOW: The Elasto-Gel Lumbar Pillow provides cold or hot therapy for the lower back. The pillow is made of contoured urethane foam for support and fitted with a gel insert. For cold treatments, pillow can be chilled in a freezer; for hot therapy, pillow can be warmed in a microwave oven. The pillow will retain the temperature for 20 to 40 minutes. The velour cover is washable and has Velcro closures. Dimensions are 14 by 13 by $3\frac{1}{2}$ inches overall; inserts are 8 by 12 inches.

PERSONAL EMERGENCY AND ALARM SYSTEMS

Colonial Medical Alert Systems, (800) 323-6794 or (603) 881-8351

MEDI-MATE: professionally monitored (operates national and local monitoring services); can be reprogrammed for alternate monitoring service; optional two-way voice.

Consumer Engineering Incorporated/Seavon Corporation, Post Office Box 060100, Palm Bay, FL 32906-0100; (407) 984-0179

911 EMERGENCY-LITE: The 911 Emergency-Lite is a strobe-light adapter designed to be placed between the bulb and socket in a regular light fixture. The adapter causes an emergency flashing light when the normal light switch is turned on twice in rapid succession.

Elcombe Systems Limited, (613) 591-5678 (Canada; all or nearest U.S. dealer)

MAINSTREET MESSENGER: Tone or digital dialer built into telephone (programmable for professional and nonprofessional monitoring); two-way voice; hands-free answering feature or regular calls with pendant.

Home Control Concepts, (800) 266-8765 or (619) 693-8887

HCC RF-1: wireless pendant with receiver; can be added to most monitored systems.

Intelecom, (405) 842-0163 or (405) 232-2809

GUARDIAN: voice dialer with pendant; dials 911 only.

Lifeline Systems, Incorporated, One Arsenal Marketplace, Watertown, MA 02172; (617) 923-4141 or (800) 451-0525

COMMUNICATION SYSTEM: Professionally monitored; two-way voice; hands-free, answer regular calls with pendant; optional smoke detector; special switches for physically challenged; rental only.

Linear Electronics, (800) 421-1587 or (619) 438-7000

ET-1B/ET-2: Wireless pendants; can be added to most monitored alarm systems; D-67: single-channel receiver.

My Alarm, (800) 235-9918 or (214) 243-7443

MY COMPANION: Telephone-based security system with voice dialer; two-way voice; variety of wireless security sensors.

Paramount, Canada, (604) 572-9588

IMEDACALL: Professionally monitored; two-way voice; rental only.

PCS, (800) 951-8733 or (910) 722-5008

CARELINE: Voice dialer with pendant; 2-way.

Protect ERS, (800) 548-8805 or (510) 671-0949

MODEL 2000AL: Professionally monitored; can be reprogrammed for alternate monitoring service.

Quorum, (800) 883-0035 or (602) 780-5500

PANIC DIALER: Voice dialer with pendant; three emergency messages; outgoing message for call screening.

Radio Shack (local stores)

AUTO DIALER 49–433: Voice dialer with panic button on console.

Telko, (714) 367-1234

EMERGENCY VOICE AUTO DIALER: Panic button on console (no pendant).

Transcience, (800) 243-3494 (203) 327-7810

RED-100: Professionally monitored; can be reprogrammed by user for alternate monitoring service; Transcience also sells components for adding a pendant to an existing alarm system.

X-10 (USA) Incorporated, (201) 784-9700

PERSONAL ALERT SYSTEM: Voice dialer with pendant; two-way voice.

WHEELCHAIRS AND WHEELCHAIR ACCESSORIES

Action Products, Incorporated, 22 N. Mulberry Street, Hagerstown, MD 21740; (800) 228-7763

Activeaid, Incorporated, One Activeaid Road, Post Office Box 359, Redwood Falls, MN 56283; (800) 533-5330

Advantage Bag Company, 22633 Ellinwood Drive, Torrance, CA 90505; (310) 540-8197

WHEELCHAIR CADDY: The down-under shelf is an under-seat carrying caddy for rigid wheelchairs designed to provide ample space for school books, shopping items, clothing, and the like; dimension 14 inches wide by 11 inches deep by 4 inches high.

WHEELCHAIR SIDE POUCH: The wheelchair side pouch is a carrying bag for wheelchairs. It is made of waterproof nylon and attaches to the inside of the wheelchair for greater security. Other features include a large main pocket, smaller pockets for wallets, checkbooks, pens, and the like, and a zipper pocket with a large zipper pull ring and tabs. It is $10^{1}/_{2}$ inches by $6^{1}/_{2}$ inches by 2 inches.

Alpha Kinetics, Incorporated, 220 Water Street West, Cannon Falls, MN 55009; (507) 263-2868

THE CRANK: The Crank is an accessory attachment for road-racing wheelchairs that allow the user to "crank" the wheels instead of pushing them. The grips eliminate the need for tape, pine tar, and full-finger gloves; only bicycle gloves are needed. The cranks have ball-bearing spindles and direct drive; there are no gears or chains. Freewheels let the cranks coast. Good for building balanced strength and no-impact, stationary roller-training. The crank will not interfere with 14-inch hand rims.

Braun Corporation, 1014 South Monticello, Post Office Box 310, Winamac, IN 46996; (219) 946-6153 or (800) 843-5449

POWER FLOOR PAN: Van floor elevator to accommodate wheelchair driver attaches to floor of van. Will lower floor up to 6 inches with self-centering toggle switch. Positions driver for proper visibility and for driving. Does not move horizontally. Individual wheel cups can also be installed in a variety of floor locations for permanent positioning of the wheelchair in the van. Will fit Ford, Chevrolet, and Dodge vans. Designed for drivers who will remain in the wheelchair. Used with a variety of other aids associated with wheelchair driving. Permanent positioning of wheelchair does not include restraint system for either wheelchair or occupant.

Car Chair Limited, 1640 Fifth Street, Suite 224, Santa Monica, CA 90401; (213) 394-3640

CAR CHAIR: Wheelchair designed to be lifted into a standard two-door car. Special lift mechanism replaces seat. Person remains seated in wheelchair during the transfer into the car, and rides in the usual front seat position, either as a passenger or driver. There are three models: powered, manually propelled, and attendant-propelled ($12\frac{1}{2}$-inch rear wheels). Solid upholstered seat and adjustable height headrest, adult size only.

Cleo, Incorporated, 3957 Mayfield Road, Cleveland, OH 44121; (216) 382-9700 or (800) 321-0595

Everest and Jennings, 1100 Corporate Square Drive, St. Louis, MO 63132-2908; (314) 569-3515 or (800) 235-4661

LANCER POWERED WHEELCHAIR: The Lancer is a powered wheelchair with a modular base for adults. The frame has a compact 24 inches wide base that accommodates the individual battery boxes. The power base measures $31^1/4$ inches long by $17^3/8$ inches tall. Minimum ground clearance is $3^1/8$ inches. Turning radius is 45 inches. The frame is available in standard black or six optional colors. Remote hand control with fuel gauge. Automatic correction for tremor in operating the joystick. Out of neutral at power up prevents the chair from starting unless the joystick is in neutral position. The standard seating is a solid seat 18 by 16 inches. Tilt-in space and recliner seating units are also available as options. A solid $1/2$-inch padded seat with sling back is standard. Options include a solid padded seat and solid back, sling seat and sling back, and van seat. Front wheels are $9^1/4$ inches; rear wheels are 12 inches in diameter. It is powered by two 24-volt batteries. A 10-amp lead acid battery charger is standard. Up to 33 miles per charge. Speeds up to 5.4 miles per hour on a 14-degree incline.

Falcon Rehabilitation Products Incorporated, 4404 East 60th Avenue, Commerce City, CO 80022; (303) 287-6808

HI-RIDER STAND UP POWERED WHEELCHAIR: The Hi-Rider is a powered stand-up wheelchair for adults designed to provide mobility in sitting and standing positions. The user can independently move to a full standing position and return to a sitting position while the chair is in a forward motion. This front-wheel drive chair is operated by a proportional joystick control. Adjustable padded leg braces and waist and chest straps stabilize user. The unit measures 41 by $22^1/2$ by 37 inches. The seat is 18 inches wide. The armrests automatically adjust when the standing feature is engaged to allow the user access to the control box. Nine-inch front wheels have electric mechanical brakes. Rear casters are 8 inches in diameter. Powered with 24-volt motors. Battery charger and tool kit are included. Maximum speed in sitting position is 5 mph; maximum speed while standing is $2^1/2$ mph for a range of 25 miles. Weight: 340 pounds.

Fortress, Incorporated, Post Office Box 489, Clovis, CA 93613-0489; (209) 323-0292 or (800) 866-4335

ACTIVE LITE, MANUAL WHEELCHAIR: Ultra lightweight manual wheelchair, folding. Weight: 27 to 29 pounds. Seat width: 16 or 18 inches. Back angle 8 inches. Various back heights available. Eight-inch front casters with semi-pneumatic tires, 24-inch rear wheels with semi-pneumatic tires or pneumatic tires, and 21-inch aluminum hand rims. Swing away, removable footrests with flip-up heel loops and 5-inch height adjustment. Removable armrests, washable, water-resistant vinyl upholstery. Optional: 8-inch front pneumatic tires, 24 by $1^1/4$-inch pneumatic rear tires, quick-release axles, plastic-coated hand rims, custom sizes, seat belt with buckle or Velcro.

BUTLER, THE LIFTING WHEELCHAIR: Power wheelchair alternative with elevating seat. High-backed padded captain's-type chair mounted on a 23- by 25-inch motorized base. Electrohydraulic cylinder lifts chair seat height from 18 to 34 inches for reaching up high while seated. Wheelchair moves forward, backward, and turns 360 degrees in place, turns right or left by activating joystick mounted on adjustable armrests. Adjustable one-piece footrest. Seat width 20.5 inches, seat depth 19.75 inches. Solid-state electronics. Power: two 12-volt batteries. Speed: high, 207 feet per minute; low, 82 feet per minute. Comments: Medicare covered with qualifications.

Fred Sammons, Incorporated, 2915 Walkent NW, Department 636, Grand Rapids, MI 49504; (616) 784-0208

Gadabout, 1165 Portland Avenue, Rochester, NY 14621; (716) 544-9060

Gendron Incorporated, 400 E. Lugbill Road, Post Office Box 197, Archibold, OH 43502; (419) 445-6060 or (800) 537-2521

SOLO II POWERED WHEELCHAIR: The Solo II is an adult folding, powered wheelchair. The overall measurement of the wheelchair is $25^1/4$ inches wide by 37 inches high by $31^1/2$ inches long. A detectable, sealed joystick is the standard controller. Full-length arms with vinyl cushion armrests, direct gear drives to slow and brake the wheelchair, standard removable footrests, detachable rear wheel hubs that permit free-wheeling are also standard. Power and speed features include: a variable-speed rotary dial, maximum speed of 5 mph, an extra-large removable battery case for storage of two deep-cycle batteries, and battery charger. This wheelchair weighs 78 pounds. Optional features include: chin control, swing away joystick, removable desk or full-length arms and accessories to fit 18- or 20-inch-wide wheelchairs.

Gunnell, Incorporated, 221 North Water Street, Vassar, MI 48768; (517) 823-8557 or (800) 551-0055

Hall's Wheels, Post Office Box 784, Cambridge, MA 02238; (617) 628-7955

Hand-crafted Metals, 13710 49th Street, North, Clearwater, FL 34622; (813) 573-2366 or (813) 526-9419

HK Enterprises, Route 6, Box 188, Bemidji, MN 56601; (218) 586-2652 or (218) 586-2419

Imex Medical, Incorporated, 5672 Almaden Expressway, San Jose, CA 95118; (408) 978-8112

Invacare Corporation, Post Office Box 4028, 899 Cleveland Street, Elyria, OH 44036-2125; (216) 329-6000 or (800) 333-6900

ROLLS ARROW POWERED RECLINER WHEELCHAIR: Powered reclining wheelchair, 16- or 18-inch seat width, 17-inch seat depth, 24-inch back height with 10-inch headrest. Power reclining backrest from 90 to 180 degrees. Leg rests elevate as back reclines. Trough-style armrests. 20-inch rear wheels with solid tires. 8-inch front casters with semi-pneumatic tires. Wheelchair and backrest can be operated by a variety of systems, including proportional or microswitch joystick, sip-n-puff, chin control, or multiple switches. Electronic brakes. Battery charger. Options: manual reclining backrest, four other arm styles, range 25 miles maximum, speed 5 miles per hour. Weight 142 pounds without batteries.

Jay Medical, Post Office Box 18656, Boulder, CO 80308-8656; (303) 442-5529 or (800) 648-8282

K-Chair Corporation, 105 W. Dakota #114, Clovis, CA 93612; (408) 243-6571

Ken Wright Supplies, Incorporated, 7456 South Oswego, Tulsa, OK 74136; (918) 492-9657

Kuschall of America, 753 Calle Plano, Camarillo, CA 93010; (805) 484-3595 or (805) 987-9844

Levo, 21050 Superior Street, Chatsworth, CA 91311; (818) 882-6944 or (800) 882-6944

Lillian Vernon, 510 South Fulton Avenue, Mount Vernon, NY 10550; (914) 633-6300

Lite-Style Wheelchair, Incorporated, Post Office Box 3926, Pinedale, CA 93650; (209) 432-1357

Magnum Poirier, One Madison Street, East Rutherford, NJ 07073; (201) 778-5585

Mobilectrics, 545 Barret Avenue, Louisville, KY 40204; (800) UR-MOVIN

Motion Designs, 2842 Business Park Avenue, Fresno, CA 93727; (209) 292-2171

Porta Ramps, 5592 East La Palma Avenue, Anaheim, CA 92807; (800) 654-7267

> PORTABLE RAMPS: The Porta Ramps are lightweight, made of maxi-strength fiberglass with nonskid full surface. Guard rails on both sides with an overall width of 30 inches and a 27-inch inside dimension (except for channel ramps). The standard one-piece ramps range in length from 3 feet to 10 feet. The folding two-piece ramps range in length from 4 feet to 14 feet. Channel ramps are sold in pairs, with lengths from 3 feet to 5 feet, with an overall width of 8 inches. Standard color is light tan. Custom-made ramps are available.

Pin Dot Products, 8100 North Austin Avenue, Morton Grove, IL 60053-9801; (708) 470-7885 or (800) 451-3553

Prime Engineering, 4838 West Jacquelyn, Suite 105, Fresno, CA 93722; (209) 276-0991

Quickie Design Incorporated, A Division of Sunrise Medical, 2842 Business Park, Fresno, CA 93727; (209) 292-2171 or (800) 456-8168

> QUICKIE P100: Powered adult wheelchair with 16- or 18-inch-width seat. Seat depth 15, 16, or 17 inches. Adjustable back height, 16 to 17, or 18 to 19 inches. 8-inch pneumatic or semi-pneumatic

front casters. 12-inch pneumatic rear wheels. 24-volt rear-wheel drive. Proportional joystick control. Lead acid or gel batteries. Battery charger. Remote-control joystick for adjustable positioning. Adjustable control parameters including acceleration, braking, and joystick sensitivity. Removable adjustable-height armrests. 8-position options including swing-away, flip-up, and adjustable-angle models. Options: backpack, wheelchair cushion, seat belt, and side guards. Assorted standard and custom frame colors. Weight, 65 pounds not including batteries. Maximum load capacity 250 pounds. Maximum speed 5 miles per hour.

Rampus Incorporated, Post Office Box 37, Coldwater, MI 49036; (800) 876-9498

FOLDING TRACKS: Portable dual tracks for wheelchair access. Nonslip material extends along entire length for tire grip. Length 3 feet. Inner channel width of each track 8 inches; 6^1/$_2$ pounds each. Maximum load capacity 550 pounds per pair.

Roho Incorporated, 100 Florida Avenue, Belleville, IL 62221-5430; (618) 277-9150 or (800) 851-3449

QUADTRO AIR CUSHION: The Quadtro cushion is designed for persons who require special positioning of the pelvis or thighs and are at risk of skin breakdown. It has a 4-inch cell height and *air in place,* which provides automatic adjustments for physiological changes as they occur. All Roho products are based on a concept of self-adjustment to the user's changing body shape, resulting in a better fit. This air cushion as well as Roho's entire product line has the ability to change a person's seated position, enhancing abilities and improving function.

Scott Orthotic Labs, 5540 Gray Street, Arvada, CO 80002; (800) 821-5795

Sears National Catalog, Home Office Department 702C-7, BSC2-14, 7447 Skokie Boulevard, Skokie, IL 60077; (708) 676-6361 or (708) 677-6326

POWERED WHEELCHAIR (MODEL 1628): Electric-powered adult, folding wheelchair. Seat width 18 inches, depth 16 inches, height 20 inches. Chrome-plated, steel frame. Arms: detachable desk length, plastic armrests, stainless-steel side panels. Footrests: hook-on detachable. Vinyl hammock seat and back upholstery. Rear-drive wheels 8 inches in diameter, semi-pneumatic. Front casters 8-inch-diameter solid tires. Control box and joystick mount on either left or right. Two 12-volt batteries. Maximum speed 3.5 mph. Batteries, power unit, and rear wheels must be removed to fold chair.

Shade and Rain Umbrella Company, Box 430, Montgomery, TX 77356; (409) 588-3415 or (409) 760-3418

Sopur West/Sunrise Medical, 566 Zinc Avenue, Santa Barbara, CA 93111-2846

ADULT LIGHTWEIGHT WHEELCHAIR: This lightweight adult wheelchair is for everyday use and weighs 29 pounds. The folding, modular frame is available in aluminum or titanium. 16 colors are available. Widths available are 12$\frac{1}{2}$ to 20 inches. The back is folding, with an adjustable-angle range of 0 to 20 degrees. The upholstery fabric is nylon or waterproof, available in 14 colors. Seat depth range is 13 to 19 inches; the standard cushion is available in 1-, 2-, or 3-inch heights, and in soft, medium, or hard foam. Coated hand rims come in 22, 24, and 26 inches. Flip-up footrests are rigid single unit, swing-away, or adjustable. Standard brakes are mid-mount; hub brakes and extension handles are available. Adjustable rubber casters are standard. Quick-release, 5- or 8- inch, and pneumatic options are available. Quick-release wheels with 20 axle positions and adjustable camber is standard, with mag wheels optional.

Theradyne Corporation, 21730 Hanover Avenue, Lakeville, MN 55044; (612) 469-4404 or (800) 328-4014

T-BIRD POWER DRIVE: Adult powered wheelchair. Black finish steel frame. Seat width 16 or 18 inches. 16-inch seat depth, 16$\frac{1}{2}$-inch back height. 24-inch rear wheels with solid tires. 8-inch solid front casters. Removable armrests. Swing-away removable footrests. 24-volt motors. Maximum speed 5.4 mph, range 12 miles. Removable power unit with proportional joystick control. Battery charger, wheel locks, seat cushion. Weight including footrests and batteries, 100 pounds.

Tumble Forms Carrie Rover, Sixty Page Road, Clifton, NJ 07012; (201) 777-2700 or (800) 631-7277

21st Century Scientific Incorporated, 4915 Industrial Way, Coeur d'Alene, ID 83814; (208) 667-8800

BIG BOUNDER—HEAVY-DUTY WHEELCHAIR: Maximum weight capacity 500 pounds. Seat width 21 inches and wider. Seat depth 15 inches and up. Swing-away removable footrests or elevating footrests. Adjustable or fixed-height desk or full-length armrests. 20-inch mag rear wheels with pneumatic tires. 8-inch front casters with pneumatic tires. 24-volt, 10-amp battery charger. Two-axis joystick proportional control, left or right side mount. Electric parking brake with automatic and manual modes. Dynamic braking. Control panel adjustments include brake duration, accelerating limiting, high- and low-speed adjustment, low-battery indicator, brake alarm, and brake holdoff.

Wheel Ring, Incorporated, 199 Forest Street, Manchester, CT 06040; (860) 647-8596

Wheelchair Carrier Company, 726 Farnsworth Road, Post Office Box 79, Waterville, OH 43566-0079; (800) 541-3213

XL Wheelchairs, 4950 D Cohasset Stage Road, Chico, CA 95926; (800) 356-3554

PART II NOTES

1. *PC Magazine*, 28 June 1994, p. 87.
2. *New Milford Times*, 8 June 1994.

Part III

Finding Help Within

Chapter • 5

Psychological Approaches

I was ten years old when the United States entered World War II in 1941. My boyhood heroes were Generals Eisenhower, MacArthur, Bradley, and Patton. Last year during the 50th anniversary of the Normandy invasion by the allied troops, I sat glued to the television set watching the reenactment and ceremonies surrounding the event. One veteran of the D-Day invasion who was interviewed as part of the celebration spoke of fear, courage, and bravery. He reminded me of the quote that my wife and I adopted at the onset of my disease, "Courage is not being without fear, but courage is to go forward in spite of fear."

I asked a good friend of mine who was severely wounded in the invasion how he felt about participating in a war knowing that he might be killed. He replied, "I always knew that someone would die in the war, but I always felt that that someone would be somebody else." When I found out that I had ALS, I discovered for myself that that "somebody else" would be me.

EMOTIONAL ADJUSTMENT

The day my disease was diagnosed, I immediately knew what my friend had meant when he spoke of courage. There was no question that I was afraid to face the future. I realized that my life had suddenly and unexpectedly taken a decisive turn. I had previously taken comfort in believing that I had at least 15 to 20 more years to live. Suddenly, 20 years became two or three.

When I arrived home that ill-fated day, I had to muster enough courage to face my wife. I tried as calmly as I could to relate to her what had taken place. When I finished, we both sat there emotionally drained. We decided to call the minister of our church, and for the next hour or two, talked about the diagnosis, the disease, and the cruelty of the situation. I don't remember what specifically was said but I do recall that when the minister left, my wife and I resolved to fight the disease and not allow it to defeat us. One advantage to having a slow progressive disease like ALS, MS, or Parkinson's is that the patient has more time to adjust to the social, emotional, physical, and overall lifestyle changes that result from the disease than a person who experiences a sudden loss from an accident or from another unforeseen event.

The initial feelings and emotions that my wife and I felt, I later read, were very similar to the feelings reported by other individuals with chronic diseases: disbelief, fear, anger, and depression. During the days immediately following my diagnosis, I also experienced a short period of fear and apprehension. I feared the uncertainty of my disease and the disabilities that would arise, and I felt apprehension about losing control over my life. I knew that my role in my family life would change and that I would no longer be the breadwinner of my household. I also realized that my role as a business executive would change as well.

You can expect that whatever your present role is, it will change, and both you and your family must learn to adjust to the situation. I believe that control over one's life is closely tied to self-image and self-respect. The more I had to relinquish, the more I had to redefine my family, social, and work relationships. I was forced to exchange my role for another one that was more helpless and dependent, but one that I knew I had to accept.

I also went through a period of grieving. After learning about the crippling nature of my disease, I couldn't help but ask myself "Why me?" Some mornings I woke up and looked out my living room window and cried, mourning the present loss and the anticipated loss of my bodily functions.

In their book *Social-Psychological Adjustment to Multiple Sclerosis, A Longitudinal Study*, Ronald Matson and Nancy Brooks[1] indicate that there are several general phases that people with chronic diseases and similar disabilities go through. They concluded, however, that not everyone experiences the same pattern of adjustment, and that effective coping does not necessarily depend on working through each of the stages. Denial, they say, is a normal reaction when a diagnosis of a disease is made. Some other reading that I have done indicates that people with chronic illnesses often use denial as a positive coping device as long as it doesn't interfere with proper treatment and self-care.[2] According to this pamphlet, "To the extent that it allows you to set aside your worries, at least for a while, [denial] can be a positive time out."

Brooks and Matson also state that patients undergo a period of resistance. While it may be helpful, they say, to take an active stance, an unrealistic expectation of your ability to conquer all may leave you dangerously open to depression and feelings of letdown if anything goes wrong.

Very soon after I was diagnosed with the disease, my wife and I began reading from a devotional book that we purchased at our neighborhood bookstore. We came across the following quote during one of our readings: "Acceptance is not defeat." Although we knew that we had to accept my disease as part of our lives, we realized that affirmation and acceptance did not mean we were defeated but only that we had come to terms with the situation. Part of the process of acceptance involves learning about how your disease can be managed. Equipped with a new realistic acceptance of the situation combined with a positive attitude, we were faced with an opportunity for our relationship to grow in new ways.

In a 1982 study by Sobel and Worden, disabled persons were asked what would make them "happy." Most of them answered that they would only be "happy" if the following conditions were met:

1. They were completely free of symptoms.

2. They were treated in the same manner they had been before they became ill.

3. They were able to do everything they did before they became ill.

4. They were no longer an inconvenience to their families.

5. They believed that their doctors were acting in their best interests.

Unfortunately, most of the above conditions are unattainable for someone with a chronic illness. More importantly, these conditions generally don't have anything to do with happiness. W. H. Auden has been quoted as saying, "To be happy means to be free, not free from pain or fear, but free from care and anxiety." Focusing our attention outside of ourselves and on hobbies, goals, and friends, for example, can give us the inspiration and enthusiasm to go forward. Accepting responsibility for our own happiness frees us from others' control.

Remember, the people who cope best with their situations are those who are actively involved in their own care, as well as in all aspects of their lives. I have always prided myself on my ability to be resourceful, optimistic, flexible, positive, and, most important, in control.

POSITIVE STRENGTH FACTORS

Many people have asked me "How is it possible to keep a positive attitude while facing an overwhelming and negative situation?" There are several factors which I believe have allowed me to not only cope with my disease but have enabled me to find new avenues for personal growth. Briefly, these positive strength factors consist of the following:

- Spiritual beliefs
- Staying in control

- Maintaining strong bonds with family and friends
- Setting goals
- Expressing concerns and feelings
- Finding a doctor with whom I feel confident and comfortable

Spiritual Beliefs

My strong religious and philosophical beliefs have helped me to understand my situation better. These deep-rooted beliefs provide me with a source of spiritual support. I believe that my faith has given me a sense of peace. This peace is not simply "peace of mind" about a troubling matter, but rather a peace that encompasses all facets of my life. It is difficult for me to explain to others exactly how I feel, but my sense of peace has given me an inner quiet, if you will, and the ability to deal with especially trying days. Individuals must reflect and dig within themselves to find their own sense of peace.

Staying in Control

Staying in control does not mean becoming (or remaining) a dictator or a tyrant. Rather, staying in control means that those with chronic illnesses or disabilities stay actively involved in the world around them, especially in their own health care. I have been able to stay in control of my life by actively participating in each phase of my situation. I continue to select doctors, evaluate treatments, volunteer in drug study programs, and actively look for ways to finance my condition.

Our lives are shaped by those who love us, those who refuse to love us, and by those who can't love us. I have found that to be loved, one must first love. I can't expect someone else to love me or even be kind to me if I'm not willing to reciprocate. In order to stay in control, one must maintain control of themselves. Don't expect others to be cheerful around you if you wallow in self-pity and are unkind to them.

A recent article in *Redbook*[3] maintains that new medical evidence points to key emotional traits that can help keep a person healthy as well as help an individual who isn't healthy cope with illness. These traits include:

- **Optimism.** Health can be a self-fulfilling prophecy, according to David Phillips, Professor of Sociology at the University of California at San Diego. Good things appear to happen to people who expect them. And, according to Michael Scheier, professor of psychology at Carnegie-Mellon University, pessimism, fatalism, and resignation have been linked to studies of poorer health.

- **Take the challenge.** The ability to treat stress or threats as a challenge rather than a negative event is a healthy approach to problems.
- **The ability to take charge.** A fighting spirit may provide the motivation to cope with a disease. Don't give up.
- **The ability to take control.** Studies of breast cancer and melanoma patients found that active copers, or those who believe they can take control of their situations, have higher survival rates.
- **A sense of humor.** "Being able to laugh at yourself—as opposed to ridiculing other people—is very health enhancing," according to Dr. Redford Williams Jr., director of the Behavioral Medicine Research Center at Duke University. Confirming this idea, Dr. Kenneth R. Pelletier, clinical associate professor at Stanford University School of Medicine, states that altruistic behavior has a physically and mentally beneficial effect. Pelletier states that his study subjects "Saw the necessity of giving back to others, making the world a better place, and doing something more than just indulging."

According to Dr. Pelletier, "If you have any of these traits you probably have another health bonus—social connectedness." A loving family and good friends can make a real difference in your health. In one Yale University study of heart attack victims, those who negatively answered to the question, "Can you count on anyone to provide you with emotional support?" were more than twice as likely to die in six months than those who said they had two or more supportive people in their lives. Beth Israel's Dr. Locke says, "The sense of being connected to other people induces biochemical changes that are probably beneficial in the healing process."

Maintaining Strong Bonds with Family and Friends

Maintaining relationships with your family and friends is an important ingredient to effective living whether you have a disability or not. Especially uplifting is the fact that I've acquired a great many new friends as a result of my disease. As social creatures, most of us need to know we are cared for and loved. We also need to be able to care for others who are important to us. When our physical capabilities change with a disabling condition, what we can do for others also changes. Discuss these changes openly with your family and friends and, together, work out new ways to maintain strong relationships. Immediately after learning about my disease, my wife and I decided to inform our family and our closest friends. We called a "family gathering" and told them what had taken place and what the future might hold. Not only did we receive full verbal support from everyone, but later we also received physical assistance and financial support. We continue to have family talk sessions where we release our feelings of anger, frustration, fear, and uncertainty. Openness and cooperation are all important to have within the family. I constantly remind myself that I am not the only one who has to adjust to my condition.

The reaction of people to a serious illness may vary tremendously. Some old friends may become uncomfortable, while others who are just acquaintances may all of a sudden become supportive friends. I've been fortunate in that very few of my old friends have disappeared.

Several months ago a friend of mine dropped by for a visit. This was a person whom I had only had a brief encounter with during the past year. After staying for an hour or so, he asked if I would mind if he came for another visit. My newly acquired friend soon visited me on a weekly basis. Another acquaintance of mine has likewise become a good friend in an entirely different way. When I purchased the electric hoist for my scooter, I had problems installing it in my station wagon. Since this acquaintance owns and operates a welding and metal fabrication company in our small town, I asked if he could assist me in installing it. When he finished the job, I asked him how much I owed. He replied, "Letting me help you with jobs like these is my way of being a friend." Since then, whenever I needed help, he was more than willing to help me in anyway possible.

I have been most fortunate in that both my newer acquaintances and friends with whom I haven't always been close and the people whom I have known for many years have provided me with support. For example, my business partner from ten years ago now meets me once a month to join him for lunch. When I was not able to drive myself, he volunteered to pick me up. And when I was no longer able to walk and needed the use of a scooter, he came to my house with his car and traded it with my car so I could fit the scooter in the back of the station wagon. Oftentimes he would also invite people that we had both worked with in the past to join us for lunch. In this way, he was keeping me actively involved with our old consulting practice.

Another individual I had worked with over 20 years ago in New Jersey called me "just to talk" upon hearing that I had health problems. He now has been calling me every three to four weeks. Both of these relationships help me keep a positive attitude.

I am most proud of my daughters and their families. They have all rallied around me and have provided strength and support whenever needed. All four of my daughters live within a $2^{1}/_{2}$-hour drive. The three that live closer come for a weekly visit, while my fourth daughter, who lives out of state, plans a weekend visit at least every six weeks and calls several times during the week. The weekly visits by my daughters are usually during the day, which gives my wife additional time to herself.

Setting Goals

If an idea I reasoned were really a valuable one, there must be some way of realizing it.

—Elizabeth Blackwell

These words were written by the first woman to earn a medical degree. It is said that you don't have to plan to climb Mount Everest in order to have a goal. I have found that having a goal—however modest—gives me something to work toward and puts some structure into my life. When I wake up in the morning, I need to be able to say to myself, "I have a purpose today." Without a specific goal for the day, I find that my day would be pointless. Goals inspire action, motivation, and exhilaration.

As I was watching the college baseball World Series games on television, a sign nailed to the back wall of the dugout caught my eye. It read, "A goal is nothing but a dream with a deadline." I have set myself a few specific goals to reach that are all realistic and obtainable. I also established a timetable to which I often refer to check the status of my progress. For example, one goal I had was to complete this book in six months. A few other of my goals are as follows:

- Study the American Civil War. This goal has forced me to visit my local library and read an enormous number of books on the subject. I have also joined a history book club where I ran into a neighbor of mine who is also a Civil War history buff.

- Return to landscape oil painting, which I stopped about two years ago. My landscape painting goal got off to a quick start only to be derailed by finally losing finger dexterity and hand strength. However, I soon discovered that I could paint almost as well with the paintbrush held in my teeth. I have thus been able to continue this project and am currently working on a covered bridge series of pictures covering the four seasons of the year.

- Work on the bicentennial committee of our church, which will be celebrating its 200th year anniversary during 1995.

- Participate in a mentoring program for middle-school students. Currently, I am working with a boy who wants to learn more about drawing and painting. My mentoring activities require the least amount of physical activity of all my projects. I include this project just to illustrate a point I made to someone a few weeks ago. I met a man at the hospital during one of my routine visits who had the same disease as I. He was quite depressed and felt that he had no reason to live. I, though, tried to convince him that regardless of his current condition, he still had something to contribute to life. By mentoring the boy who wanted to learn to draw and paint, I am able to pass on to him some experience I've acquired. No one can say to a disabled person that he or she has no talent. For instance, people who have lost the use of all their body movements but still have their sight and voices can read for the blind. The man I previously discussed, although totally paralyzed, is able to write poetry by blinking his eyelids.

Keep in mind that establishing goals provides people with chronic illnesses a real sense of purpose and a means of coping with their conditions. It also forces disabled persons to interact with people and have some direction in their lives.

Expressing Concerns and Feelings

It is important to have at least one trusted individual with whom you can talk about how your illness or injury is affecting your life. If you feel this would be a burden to relatives and friends, get in touch with a pastor or counselor or even your local Volunteer Association (refer to the listing at the end of this section). Most people find that talking with someone from time to time lets off steam, provides perspective, and reduces tension.

One person I have found who is able to understand what I am feeling and thinking is a person I met six years ago who was told he was dying of cancer. He experienced all of the same feelings that I did such as denial, resentment, anger, bewilderment, fear, and acceptance. I have been able to share both my successes and failures with him. In 1986, my friend underwent surgery and chemotherapy and is currently celebrating his ninth cancer-free year. His experience with the disease has inspired me to find direction in my own life.

Besides the importance of communicating with people, what you "say" to yourself each day is also significant. Shifting from saying "This situation is impossible" to "I think I can handle this" is a major step towards a healthier life. In a recent health column, "Health Notes," Dr. Peter Gott[4] puts a different slant on "attitude adjustment." He built his column around a children's fable called "Nail Broth." In this simple story, a tramp attempts to obtain lodging and supper from a suspicious and stingy old lady. She gives him a place to rest in the barn but refuses him any food since she claims she doesn't have enough to spare.

The tramp offers to make a cheap supper for both of them by boiling a four-inch nail in a pot of water. After a few minutes, the tramp acknowledges that the concoction is a little thin but suspects that a handful of flour would thicken it. She reluctantly obliges and ends up adding salt beef, potatoes, barley, and milk to the supper. Eventually the broth is ready to eat. The old woman who has been so caught up in the charade sets the table and supplies enough food for a feast. The next morning after allowing him to stay the night, she gives the tramp breakfast and money and sends him on his way, praising him for making such a delicious broth from just an old nail.

Choosing to ignore the obvious "lesson" of the story, Dr. Gott implies that the real worthwhile message here is that unpleasant situations can be modified and made palatable. In real life, for example, he says that the threat of major illnesses, diseases, and catastrophic injuries can be ameliorated by methods that reduce fear and uncertainty. Although the nail broth is a nutrition-free scam, good ingredients can transform it into a hearty meal. To a large extent, each of us has a responsibility to each other. That responsibility may be to add a little joy, humor, caring, and affection to the nail broth we all face every day.

Being Comfortable with Your Physician

Any doctor can prescribe medication and give you periodic examinations. But having a physician whom you respect and with whom you feel comfortable discussing important health matters can make a big difference in your overall well-being and in how successful you are able to cope with your illness.

Depending on the nature of the disability, the patient generally has two physicians: a family physician (who may be an internist, family practitioner, or general practitioner) and a specialist (such as a neurologist, orthopedic surgeon, or rehabilitation specialist). The specialist often makes the diagnosis, or confirms the diagnosis of the family doctor, while the family doctor treats the patient over the length of the illness in conjunction with the specialist. Because most disabilities we are discussing are either chronic conditions or permanent disabilities, the physician you choose should be one with whom you feel personally comfortable. When choosing a doctor consider the following:

- How much does the doctor know about your particular physical problem? How many other similar patients has he or she treated?
- Is this doctor able and willing to give supportive care for a long time?
- Is the doctor willing to cooperate with another physician (the specialist) in long-term care?
- Are the doctor and the specialist willing to communicate with you; that is, are both of them willing to answer your questions or do they tend to "put you off"?

Although you may not want to know everything about your disease, injury, or illness, you should feel satisfied with the doctor's answers to your questions. A vague feeling that the doctor is not telling you the whole story often leads to disgust later. Let me give you a specific example. One of the examinations I underwent required that a blunt instrument be run along the sole of my foot. I asked the doctor what this examination was for and he gave me a vague, unsatisfactory answer. This led me to stop by my local library and do a little research.

I discovered much more than I really wanted to know at that time. Since this incident, I never fully trusted that doctor again and later decided to find another physician. Keep in mind that distrust in your doctor can lead to a failure to follow prescribed treatments or a failure to notify your doctor of important changes in symptoms.

- Does the specialist object to you getting second opinions? The diagnosis of diseases such as ALS, MS, Parkinson's disease, and similar diseases takes time to reach, and after careful and exhaustive testing, even expert neurologists can misdiagnose these diseases on rare occasions. Since the consequence of having these diseases often involves significant lifestyle changes, you should make sure that the diagnosis is accurate. Most specialists recognize this and encourage patients to get second opinions. You owe it to yourself to get the care that you personally feel comfortable with; this feeling of comfort often begins with the belief that the specialist is competent and is being honest with you.

- Do the specialist and the family doctor have good rapport with the other members of the health care team? This "team" consists of nurses, therapy specialists, social workers and aides. The physicians are usually regarded as the captains of the team; however, no team functions well if the captain does not have a good working relationship with the "crew." If at times it becomes apparent that certain team members are not performing to your satisfaction, you should ask that changes be made.

EMOTIONAL SUPPORT PROFESSIONALS

Not everyone is able to deal with disability problems by themselves. Some patients and their caregivers may need additional help in dealing with the necessary emotional adjustments. Some of the signs that should be recognized include: a failure of the patient and the caregiver to communicate each other's needs; a tendency for small problems to go unresolved; an increase in symptoms such as headaches related to "tension"; and a general sense that the situation is overwhelming. Some professional and peer support groups available include:

Psychologists and Psychiatrists

A psychiatrist is a physician who specializes in treating emotional problems through the use of psychotherapy, medication, or both. A clinical psychologist can give advice on dealing with emotional problems but cannot prescribe medication. Either of these two professionals may be able to give individual help if you are having difficulty in adjusting to your disabling problem. Keep in mind that psychotherapy is based on the assumption that a person will choose to change. According to an article by Judith C. MacNutt,[5] a practicing psychotherapist, this doesn't always happen. She says that studies show that one-third of the people undergoing psychiatric care show improvement while the other two-thirds either refuse to change their attitudes toward life or simply find themselves incapable of making the necessary changes.

If other areas of counseling and emotional support fail, you should ask your family doctor or your specialist for a referral rather than try to find a psychiatrist or psychologist yourself. Beware of self-styled psychiatrists and "faith healers," who are all too ready to "treat" patients with chronic diseases.

Clergy

I have personally found that the clergy are usually ready, willing, and able to provide spiritual as well as physical assistance and guidance. As I mentioned previously, the first person that my wife and I called after receiving my diagnosis was the minister of our church. Ministers are educated and trained to provide counseling services to persons who have just had "emotional train wrecks." In the first few hours after our "train wreck," our minister helped us sort out our feelings and fears. She helped us focus on the immediate future and how we were going to handle things like informing our family and getting second opinions.

Also, ministers usually have direct connections with support services, nursing help, food banks, and hospice organizations. In addition, almost every church or synagogue has some type of "emergency funding" available which the minister or rabbi can use for specific needs.

Support Groups

A group of people sharing a similar problem often can be helpful to a person who has newly discovered that he or she has that same problem. Members of a support group can often pass onto other members their experiences in a meaningful way. Support groups are composed of patients, family members, and caregivers and are under the direction of experienced leaders. They are a source of renewal and strength. I sincerely hope that the use of this book can supplement your finding a strong support group in your community. Almost every volunteer health agency has affiliated support groups in cities and states across the country. Some support groups are part of a chapter network while others are independent groups that fall under the auspices of national offices. Refer to the resource listing at the end of this section for a listing of volunteer health agencies.

Social Workers

While social workers may offer counseling, they do not directly attend to any of the patient's physical needs. This health care professional, though, is important in providing the patient contacts with many other professional helpers. Social workers often know people who work in service agencies and in hospital counseling services. In addition, they are often members of a voluntary health organization's paid staff. Using a variety of contacts, the social worker can help the patient reach competent professional and peer helpers. In addition, a social worker who holds an M.S.W. degree has had training in psychotherapy and in group and family counseling. If you have a good relationship with a social worker, you may want to go to this professional for help in dealing with emotional adjustments to your particular problems.

It is important to emphasize one point here: You are ultimately responsible for meeting your needs. You can meet this responsibility by making your needs known as early as possible and as clearly as possible. Although social workers, clergy, friends, neighbors, and health care professionals are all available to help you, you ultimately must help yourself. Because most of the professional helpers I have discussed are part of large health care systems, you sometimes have to be persistent in making your needs known. If your needs are refused or ignored, keep trying until your needs are met.

Other Resources

VOLUNTEER HEALTH AGENCIES

The following pages contain information about five voluntary health agencies. These agencies are operated for the sole purpose of providing assistance to individuals suffering from the designated illnesses, injuries, and diseases. They are good advocates and, in some cases, excellent sources of medical expense funding.

The Muscular Dystrophy Association, 3300 East Sunrise Drive, Tucson, AZ 85718-3208; (800) 572-1717

> The Muscular Dystrophy Association is a voluntary health agency consisting of scientists and concerned citizens organized to conquer neuromuscular diseases. There are over 189 local MDA offices available to help anyone with one of the 40 neuromuscular diseases in the Association's program, regardless of the person's ability to pay. The following is a brief recap of the activities this organization sponsors. For more information refer to the handbook *MDA Services for the Individual, Family and Community* or the "Muscular Dystrophy Association 1994 Fact Sheet."[6]

Network of Clinics	There are over 240 MDA hospital-affiliated clinics nationwide which provide diagnostic services and therapeutic and rehabilitative follow-up care. These clinics sponsor support groups and physical therapy sessions. They also assist patients in purchasing and repairing wheelchairs. Social service and genetic counseling are also available.
Summer Camps	MDA provides summer camping activities geared to the special needs of children with neuromuscular diseases.

Professional and Public Health Education

Knowledge and awareness of neuromuscular disease is furthered by MDA-sponsored scientific publications dealing with neuromuscular disease. International scientific meetings on neuromuscular research are held as well as conferences given by MDA clinic directors and their associates.

Through the help of grants and fellowships, the MDA is also promoting international research groups that seek cures for the 40 neuromuscular disorders in the MDA program. By calling the toll-free telephone number listed on the previous page, you can obtain the number and location of the nearest MDA office.

The National Multiple Sclerosis Society, 733 Third Avenue, New York, NY 10017-3278; (800) LEARN MS

The National Multiple Sclerosis Society is the only national voluntary health agency that supports national and international research into the cause, prevention, and cure of multiple sclerosis.

This society has more than 32,000 members nationwide in over 140 chapters and branches throughout the United States. Policies and goals are developed by the National Board of Directors consisting of outstanding leaders in the business and professional world, as well as individuals with a personal interest in MS.

Multiple sclerosis is a chronic disease of the central nervous system in which simple, everyday tasks can no longer be taken for granted. The 140 branches and chapters help people with MS meet the challenges of life after diagnosis. By contacting the National Office listed above, a patient or the patient's family will be put in touch with a chapter or branch of the society nearest their home.

The National Multiple Sclerosis Society has programs and activities organized into the following four major areas:

- Research to find the cause of the disease and to explore methods of preventing its onset, alleviating its symptoms, and halting its progression.
- Service at the community level for persons with MS and their families.
- Support of local and national legislation to improve the quality of life for people with MS.

- Mobilization of volunteers and public and private funds in support of these goals.

   In addition to the previous goals and objectives, the local branches and chapter programs provide support, therapy, professional and public education, literature, equipment, and emergency medical assistance.

The National Head Injury Foundation, 1776 Massachusetts Avenue NW, Suite 100, Washington, DC 20036-1904; (202) 296-6443

   The National Head Injury Foundation is also known in some states as the Traumatic Brain Injury Association (TBIA). As a not-for-profit agency working for individuals with traumatic brain injury, these associations . . .

- Promote support groups and service systems for survivors and their families.
- Educate the public about traumatic brain injuries, the related problems, and prevention.
- Advocate community and medical resources needed to provide comprehensive TBI care.
- Directly meet selected needs that are currently not addressed by existing systems.

   It is estimated that medical technology now saves 60 to 70 percent of victims who previously would have died from traumatic brain injury. These survivors now constitute a new group of people needing help. A survivor of traumatic brain injury typically faces five to ten years of intensive services, and only 1 survivor of a head injury in 20 receives appropriate rehabilitation.[7]

Arthritis Foundation, Post Office Box 19000, Atlanta, GA 30326; (800) 283-7800

   The Arthritis Foundation is a national nonprofit organization whose mission is to: "Support research to find the cure and prevention of arthritis and to improve the quality of life for those affected by arthritis."

   There are over 70 chapters of the foundation nationwide which provide a ready resource for people with arthritis. It is felt that education is the first step in controlling arthritis, and to this end, the foundation provides a wide range of programs and services, such as the following:

Arthritis Self-help Course	Teaches persons with arthritis to take an active role in the management of arthritis through education, information sharing, and demonstration.
Arthritis P.A.C.E. (People with Arthritis Can Exercise) Program	Improves physical and mental well-being through group exercise and activity.
Arthritis Foundation YMCA Aquatic Program	Helps improve joint function with specially designed exercises in a warm-water pool.
Arthritis Support Group Network	An ongoing education, information, and mutual support group.
Jerry Walsh Direct Assistance Program	Provides financial assistance for the purchase of self-help devices.

The ALS Association, 21021 Ventura Boulevard, Suite 321, Woodland Hills, CA 91364; (818) 340-7500 or (800) 782-4747

The ALS Association is the only national nonprofit voluntary health organization dedicated solely to the fight against ALS through research, patient support, information dissemination, and public awareness. While working to discover the cause, prevention, and cure for ALS, the Association is also committed to enhancing the quality of life for ALS patients and their families.

The ALS Association was formed through the merger of the ALS Society of America and the National ALS Foundation in 1985. As a single, unified national organization, the ALS Association is able to provide a powerful impetus toward the attainment of their objectives.

The ALS Association programs are supported entirely by volunteers. The association receives no government grants, nor does it seek or receive fees from patients and their families. The ALS Association provides funds both for research and for patient care through more than 100 chapters and support groups across the country.

VOLUNTARY ORGANIZATIONS FOR THE DISABLED

The following is only a partial listing of voluntary organizations dedicated to the research and cure of specific diseases, injuries, or congenital defects, and to helping people who suffer from them. This listing is not intended to be comprehensive, but is only an indicator of what is available. To use this list effectively, you should first call the telephone number listed and ask for any written material available. If you desire to reach additional agencies, refer to the *Encyclopedia of Associations,* which can be found at any public library. Your local telephone directory is also a good source for locating local associations dedicated to the particular disability that is of interest to you.

Alcoholism

American Society of Addiction Medicine–
Substance Abuse
5225 Wisconsin Avenue NW
Suite 409
Washington, DC 20015
(202) 244-8948

Alcoholics Anonymous World Service
475 Riverside Drive
New York, NY 10163
(212) 870-3400

National Council on Alcoholism
12 West 21st Street
New York, NY 10010
(212) 206-6770

Amputation

American Orthotic and Prosthetic
Association
1650 Kings Street, Suite 500
Alexandria, VA 22314
(703) 836-7116

National Amputation Foundation
12–45 150th Street
Whitestone, NY 11357
(718) 767-0596

Ataxia

National Ataxia Foundation
750 Twelve Oaks Center
15500 Wayzata Boulevard
Wayzata, MN 55371
(612) 473-7666

Birth Defects

American Genetic Association
Post Office Box 39
Buckleystown, MD 21717-0039
(301) 695-9292

Rubinstein-Toybi Parent Group
414 East Kansas
Smith Center, KS 66967
(913) 282-6237

Blindness, Visual Impairment

American Council of the Blind
1155 15th Street NW, Suite 720
Washington, DC 20005
(202) 467-5081

National Association for Visually
Handicapped
22 West 21st Street
New York, NY 10010
(212) 889-3141

National Eye Research Foundation
c/o Pamela Baker
910 Skokie Boulevard, No. 207A
Northbrook, IL 60062
(708) 564-4652

Blood Disorders

American Society of Hematology
1101 Connecticut Avenue NW, 7th Floor
Washington, DC 20036
(202) 857-1118

Leukemia Society of America
600 Third Avenue
New York, NY 10016
(212) 573-8484

Brain Damage

National Foundation for Brain Research
1250 24th NW, Suite 300
Washington, DC 20037
(202) 293-5453

Institutes for the Achievement
of Human Behavior
Post Office Box 7226
Stafford, CA 94309
(415) 851-8411

Burn Injuries

American Burn Association
Baltimore Regional Burn Center
Francis Scott Key Hospital
4940 Eastern Avenue
Baltimore, MD 21224
(800) 548-2876

National Fire Protection Association
One Batterymarch Park
Post Office Box 9101
Quincy, MA 02269
(617) 770-3000

National Institute for Burn Medicine
909 East Ann Street
Ann Arbor, MI 48104l
(313) 769-9000

Cancer

American Association for Cancer
Research
Institute for Cancer Research
620 Chestnut Street, Suite 816
Philadelphia, PA 19106
(215) 440-9300

American Cancer Society,
1599 Clifton Road NE
Atlanta, GA 30320
(404) 320-3333

National Cancer Foundation
1180 Avenue of the Americas
New York, NY 10036
(212) 221-3300

Cardiac Disorders

American College of Cardiology
9111 Old Georgetown Road
Bethesda, MD 20814
(301) 897-5400

American Heart Association
7272 Greenville Avenue
Dallas, TX 75231-4596
(214) 373-6300

Heart Disease Research Foundation
50 Court Street, Room 306
Brooklyn, NY 11201
(718) 649-6210

Cerebral Palsy

American Academy for Cerebral Palsy
and Developmental Medicine
1910 Byrd Avenue, Suite 100
Post Office Box 11086
Richmond, VA 23230-1086
(804) 282-0036

United Cerebral Palsy Associations
1522 K Street NW, Suite 1112
Washington, DC 20005
(202) 842-1266

Cystic Fibrosis

Cystic Fibrosis Foundation
6931 Arlmston Road No. 200
Bethesda, MD 20814
(301) 951-4422

Diabetes

American Diabetes Association
Post Office Box 25757
1660 Duke Street
Alexander, VA 22314
(703) 549-1500

Joslin Diabetes Foundation
Incorporated
One Joslin Place
Boston, MA 02215
(617) 732-2400

Disfigurement

American Society of Plastic and
Reconstructive Surgeons
444 East Algonquin Road
Arlington Heights, IL 60005
(708) 228-9900

Epilepsy

American Epilepsy Society
630 Prospect Avenue
Hartford, CT 06105
(860) 232-4825

Epilepsy Foundation of America
4351 Garden City Drive
Landover, MD 20705
(301) 453-3700

Hearing Disorders

American Speech and Hearing Association
10801 Rockville Place
Rockville, MD 20852
(301) 887-5700

National Association of the Deaf
814 Thayer Avenue
Silver Spring, MD 20910
(301) 587-1788

Deafness Research Foundation
9 East 38th Street, 7th Floor
New York, NY 10016
(212) 684-6556

Kidney Disease

American Society for Artificial Internal
Organs
Box C
Boca Raton, FL 33432
(407) 319-8589

National Kidney Foundation
30 East 33rd Street, Suite 1100
New York, NY 10016
(212) 883-2210

Medic-Alert Organ Donor Program
2323 Colorado Avenue
Turlock, CA 95380
(209) 668-3333

Learning Disabilities

Association for Childhood Education
International
11501 Georgia Avenue, Suite 312
Wheaton, MD 20902
(301) 942-2443

National Association of State
Directors of Special Education
1800 Diagonal Road, Suite 320
Alexandria, VA 22314
(703) 519-3800

Leprosy

American Leprosy Missions
1 ALM Way
Greenville, SC 29601
(803) 271-7040

Leonard Wood Memorial for the
Eradication of Leprosy
11600 Noble Street, Suite 210
Rockville, MD 20852
(301) 984-1336

Mental Illness

American Academy of Psychoanalysis
47 East 19th Street, 6th Floor
New York, NY 10003
(212) 475-7980

American Psychiatric Association
1400 K Street NW
Washington, DC 20005
(202) 682-6000

American Mental Health Foundation
2 East 86th Street
New York, NY 10028
(212) 737-9027

Mental Retardation

American Academy on Mental Retardation
c/o Jack Stark, Ph.D.
Creighton-Nebraska University
Department of Psychiatry
2205 South 10th Street
Omaha, NE 68108
(402) 449-4783

Orthopedic Disorders

American Osteopathic Association
6300 North River Road, Suite 300
Rosemont, IL 60018-4263
(703) 318-7330

Association of Bone and Joint
Surgeons
6300 North River Road, Suite 727
Rosemont, IL 60018-4226
(708) 698-1628

Parkinson's Disease

American Parkinson Disease Association
60 Bay Street, Suite 401
Stanton, NY 10301
(718) 981-8081

National Parkinson Foundation
1501 Northwest Ninth Avenue
Miami, FL 33136
(305) 537-6666

United Parkinson Foundation
360 West Superior Street
Chicago, IL 60610
(312) 664-2344

Pulmonary Disorders

Allergy Foundation of America
1125 15th Street NW, Suite 502
Washington, DC 20005
(202) 466-7643

American Lung Association
1740 Broadway
New York, NY 10019
(212) 315-8700

Speech Disorders

Academy of Aphasia
c/o Dr. Victoria L. Franklin
UCLA Department of Linguistics
Los Angeles, CA 90024
(310) 206-3206

American Cleft Palate Association
1218 Grand View Avenue
Pittsburgh, PA 15211
(412) 481-1376

American Speech and Hearing
Association
10801 Rockville Place
Rockville, MD 20852
(301) 897-5700

Spina Bifida

Spina Bifida Association of America
4590 MacArthur Boulevard NW, Suite 250
Washington, DC 20007
(202) 944-3285

Spinal Cord Injury

National Spinal Cord Injury Association
600 West Cummings Park, Suite 2000
Woburn, MA 01801
(617) 935-2722

Stroke

Stroke Clubs International America
805 12th Street
Galveston, TX 77550
(409) 762-1022

PART III NOTES

1. N. Brooks and R. Matson, *Social-Psychological Adjustment to Multiple Sclerosis: A Longitudinal Study* (1982).

2. M.E. Sanford and J.H. Petajan, "Multiple Sclerosis and Your Emotions" (Provo: Multiple Sclerosis Clinic, Department of Neurology, University of Utah School of Medicine, 1989).

3. Catherine Clifford, *Redbook* (January 1995).

4. Peter Gott, M.D., "Health Notes," *The Register Citizen,* Torrington and Winsted, CT, 19 February 1995.

5. Judith C. MacNutt, *Weavings* 4, no. 4 (July/August 1991).

6. "Muscular Dystrophy Association 1994 Fact Sheet" and *MDA Services for the Individual, Family and Community.*

7. Statistics from the Interagency Head Injury Task Force Report (National Institute of Neurological Disorders and Stroke, National Institute of Health) Washington, D.C.

Money
Matters

Chapter • 7

Financial Help

Often, the most immediate issue for someone who is disabled is how to put financial affairs in order. Special arrangements may need to be made in order to ensure that care is adequate. You may need to turn to others to get the financial advice you need.

PROFESSIONAL ADVOCATES

Lawyers

Lawyers are well equipped to assist you in solving many of your financial problems. However, attorney fees can be quite exorbitant for those on fixed incomes. I was able to reduce my fees greatly by working out a plan with my attorney, whereby I did all of the legwork, such as making telephone calls and writing letters. My attorney then advised me over the telephone at a highly reduced rate. In this fashion, I was able to act on good, sound legal advice without accumulating enormous legal bills. Some subjects that my attorney assisted me with are the following:

- Wills for both me and my wife
- Living wills
- Durable power of attorney
- Designation of health care agent

Without going into a long discussion about wills (except to note that you should have one), I think that it would be beneficial to discuss living wills, durable power of attorney, and appointment of a health care agent. These three legal documents are referred to as "advance directives," that is, future health care alternative decisions that may have to be made prior to your death. If you are not able to make health care decisions for yourself at some point in the future, the living will and the durable power of attorney spell out who will make these decisions for you. If you do not have these documents in place now, you should consider doing so immediately . It is not necessary to have a lawyer draw them up. If you have any questions regarding the living will statutes in your state, your local legal aid society or your area's agency on aging are two good information sources. To obtain assistance in locating preprinted living will forms for your state, contact the following:

Choice in Dying
250 West 57th Street
New York, NY 10107
(212) 246-6962
(specify which state form you want)

The living will is a document in which you explain your desires concerning the use of medical procedures that extend the dying process and sustain life. It is used to detail the circumstances in which you would rather not continue living. A typical living will form is shown on the following page.

In most states, living wills become effective when the signer is considered to be terminally ill or permanently unconscious. The living will tells your physician whether you want life support systems to keep you alive in these situations or whether you do not want to receive treatment, even if the result is death. A living will goes into effect only when: (1) you are unable to make or communicate your decisions about your medical care, and (2) when you are in a terminal condition or become permanently unconscious.

A patient is in a "terminal condition" when the physician finds that the patient has a condition that is incurable or irreversible and will result in death within a relatively short time if life support systems are not provided. "Permanently unconscious" refers to a permanent state of coma or a persistent vegetative state in which the patient is not aware of self or surroundings and is unresponsive.

A life support system is a form of treatment that only delays the time of your death or maintains you in a state of permanent unconsciousness. Life support systems may include:

- Devices such as respirators and dialysis
- Cardiopulmonary resuscitation (CPR)
- Food and liquids supplied by artificial means, such as feeding tubes and intravenous fluids. It does not include normal feeding and fluids, such as by hand or straw.
- Medications such as antibiotics

In most states, two witnesses must sign a living will and have their signatures notarized. The declarant of the living will may change the will at any time.

Document Concerning Withholding or Withdrawal of Life Support Systems

If the time comes when I am incapacitated to the point when I can no longer actively take part in decisions for my own life and am unable to direct my physician as to my own medical care, I wish this statement to stand as a testament of my wishes. I, _____, request that, if my condition is deemed terminal, or if I am determined to be permanently unconscious, I be allowed to die and not be kept alive through life support systems. By "terminal condition," I mean that I have an incurable or irreversible medical condition which, without the administration of life support systems, will, in the opinion of my attending physician, result in death within a relatively short time. By "permanently unconscious" I mean that I am in a permanent coma or persistent vegetative state, which is an irreversible condition in which I am at no time aware of myself or the environment and show no behavioral response to the environment. The life support systems which I do not want include, but are not limited to:

___ Artificial respiration

___ Cardiopulmonary resuscitation

___ Artificial means of providing nutrition and hydration

(Cross out and initial life support systems you want administered)

I do not intend any direct taking of my life, but only that my dying not be unreasonably prolonged.

Other requests:

This request is made, after careful reflection, while I am of sound mind.

Signature_____ Date_____

This document was signed in our presence, by the above-named who appeared to be eighteen years of age or older, of sound mind, and able to understand the nature and consequences of health care decisions at the time the document was signed.

Executed at_____,

this day of_____, 19___.

Witness_____ Address_____

Witness_____ Address_____

A power of attorney is a written document in which you appoint another person or institution to act on your behalf. The most common power of attorney found in my home state of Connecticut is known as the "Statutory Short Form Power of Attorney." This type of form allows you to authorize an "attorney-in-fact" to act as your agent with respect to banking transactions, real estate transactions, business matters, and a host of other matters. It is not necessary to have an attorney draft a basic durable power of attorney form. Some states supply a "fill-in-the-blank" type of form. If you do not want to use your state's form, treat it as a guide when writing your own version.

Keep in mind that not all powers of attorney are "durable." For the power of attorney to be durable, it must contain these words:

> This power of attorney shall not be affected by the subsequent
> disability or incompetence of the principal.

If a power of attorney does not have these words or similar words, it will stop being effective if and when you, the principal, become incompetent.

Most states have added health care decisions to the list of matters that you can delegate by the power of attorney. Usually the power of attorney will not automatically authorize the attorney-in-fact to withdraw life support systems. Thus, it is necessary for you to execute a living will specifying what you want done by your agent or attorney-in-fact. A durable power of attorney becomes effective when you sign it and may be revoked by you at any time. There are two key features of the durable power of attorney:

- It allows the signer to name trusted individuals to be agents and make decisions or choices on behalf of the signer in the event the signer becomes incompetent or incapable.

- It is more flexible and broader than the living will. If you use your state's preprinted living will form, it can be enhanced with a durable power of attorney, which may contain instructions on matters not covered by the preprinted form.

In the durable power of attorney, you can explain exactly what you mean by "being allowed to die with dignity," or by not wanting to be a "burden to anyone." It will also be used by your health care agents when and if they need to decide if you should continue living.

In addition to the living will and the durable power of attorney, my wife and I both executed documents that specifically appoint both a primary health care agent and a secondary health care agent. A sample copy of this document that follows:

Document Concerning the Appointment of Health Care Agent

I appoint_____, of_____, to be my health care
agent. If my attending physician determines that I am unable to understand
and appreciate the nature and consequences of health care decisions and to
reach and communicate an informed decision regarding treatment, my health
care agent is authorized to:

1. Convey to my physician my wishes concerning the withholding or
   removal of life support systems.

2. Take whatever actions are necessary to ensure that my wishes are given
   effect.

If this person is unwilling or unable to serve as my health care agent, I
appoint_____, of_____, to be my alternative health care
agent.

This request is made, after careful reflection, while I am sound of mind.

Signature_____ Date_____

This document was signed in our presence, by the above-named who appeared
to be eighteen years of age or older, of sound mind, and able to understand the
nature and consequences of health care decisions at the time the document
was signed.

Executed at _____,

this_____ day of_____, 19___.

Witness _____ Address _____

Witness _____ Address _____

It has also been suggested in some material on durable power of attorney
instructions that it may be worthwhile to consult an elder law attorney by contacting your local bar association, your state agency on aging, or:

National Academy of Elder Law Attorneys
655 North Alvernon Way, Suite 108
Tucson, AZ 85711
(602) 881-4005

It is also recommended that copies of the durable power of attorney be given to everyone who has responsibilities for your health care such as:

- Your physician
- The person or persons you have named as a health care agent or as your attorney-in-fact for health care decisions
- Anyone who will make the existence of your advance directives known if you cannot do so yourself, such as family members, close friends, and your lawyer

You should bring copies of the durable power of attorney when you are admitted to a hospital, nursing home, or other health care facility so that it becomes part of your medical record.

Independent Living Advocates

When I decided to purchase a stair lift, I searched for possible financial sources. I was given the name of two organizations here in Connecticut that could assist me. While one is strictly a state agency, the second is associated with a national organization dedicated to providing information, support, and guidance for persons who are disabled and need help to reach their goals of independent living. The Centers for Independent Living referred me to a "personal advocate" who was extremely helpful and knowledgeable with regard to agencies that could help me. During the first year after my diagnosis, I found that just having someone to talk to about the bureaucratic red tape and the "that's not my job" syndrome was extremely comforting.

The Centers for Independent Living are unique in several ways:

- They are directed, managed, and staffed by qualified persons with severe disabilities. Many of these people have experienced discrimination firsthand and are committed to gaining independent living for all individuals.
- Most services are directed by the requirements of the consumer.
- They promote positive changes in the community through education and advocacy.
- Center services are based in the community. In Connecticut, for example, there are five centers located in major metropolitan areas.

Some services provided by most Centers for Independent Living are peer counseling and independent-living skills training. Also, these centers usually provide services to the community in the form of disability-awareness programs.

For a listing of Independent Living Centers in your area contact the following:

ILRU Research and Training Center on Independent Living at TIRR
3233 Weslayan, Suite 100
Houston, TX 77027
(713) 960-9961 or TDD (713) 960-0145

SOCIAL SECURITY DISABILITY BENEFITS

Social Security Disability Benefits are cash disability benefits paid to persons who are unable to work for a year or more because of their disability. The Social Security Administration (SSA) defines *disability* as the state of being unable to do any kind of work for which you are suited. This inability to work must be expected to last for at least one year or expected to result in death. Social Security Disability benefits continue until the disabled person is able to work again on a regular basis, dies, or reaches retirement age, at which time the payments continue as retirement benefits. These benefits are available to people at any age and to certain members of the disabled person's family. As detailed in the Social Security Administration publication titled *Disability*,[1] the disabled person's family includes:

- An unmarried son or daughter, including a stepchild, adopted child, or in some cases, a grandchild. The child must be under 18 or under 19 if in high school full-time.

- An unmarried son or daughter, 18 or over, if he or she has a disability that started before the age of 22.

- A spouse who is 62 or older.

- A spouse at any age if he or she is caring for a child of the disabled individual who is under 16 or disabled and also receiving disability benefits.

To qualify for Social Security benefits, you must have worked long enough and recently enough in Social Security–covered work. In general terms, however, you earn up to a maximum of four credits per year based on your earnings for that year.

You may request a Social Security Disability application in person at your local SSA office or by mail or telephone. Since there is usually a waiting period of six months, you should file an application as soon as you become disabled. The claims process for disability benefits is longer than other Social Security benefit applications since it takes longer to obtain the necessary medical information and to assess your disability and capability to work. For instance, it took me over 90 days from when I first applied to receive my first disability check.

When you apply for benefits, you should have the following documents ready:

- Your Social Security number and proof of age for each person applying for payments.
- Names and addresses of all doctors, hospitals, and institutions that treated you and the dates of treatment.
- A summary of where you worked in the past 15 years and what position you held.
- A copy of your W-2 Form or your federal tax return for the past year.

Your medical records, obtained from your doctor or hospital where treatment was provided, will be reviewed by a team of physicians and disability evaluation specialists. These individuals from the Disability Determination Services Office in your state will consider all the facts and decide if you are disabled. If all the medical information required by the evaluation team is not available, you may be asked to take a special examination. Once a decision is made on your claim, you will receive a written "Notice of Award." If your claim is approved you will be shown the amount of your benefits and when the payments will begin. If your claim is not approved, you will be told why. If your claim is denied, you may file an appeal. Your local SSA office will assist you in preparing the appeals paperwork.

The amount of your Social Security Disability Benefits is based on your lifetime average earnings covered by Social Security. An estimate of your disability benefits can be obtained through your local SSA office or by calling (800) 772-1213. Remember, your benefits will continue as long as you are disabled. You will, however, be reviewed periodically to determine if you are still disabled. These reviews can be as frequent as six to eighteen months if medical improvement is expected, or as long as seven years if medical improvement is not expected.

You will automatically be enrolled in Medicare once you receive disability benefits for two years. Medicare, Medicaid, and Medigap will be covered in detail later in this chapter.

Lastly, Social Security has developed "work incentives," which encourage disabled individuals to return to work. For example:

- **Trial Work Period.** For nine months (not necessarily consecutive), you can earn as much as you can without affecting your benefits. A trial work month is one in which you earn more than $200. After the trial work period is completed, your work is evaluated to see if it is "substantial." If your earnings do not average more than $500 a month, benefits will continue. If the earnings average more than $500 per month, benefits will continue for three additional months before they stop.

- **Extended Period of Eligibility.** For 36 months after a successful trial work period, if you are still disabled, you will be eligible for monthly benefit payments any month your earnings drop below $500.
- **Deductions for Impairment-Related Expenses.** Work expenses related to your disability will not be included in your gross earnings when figuring whether your earnings are "substantial."
- **Medicare Continuation.** Medicare coverage will continue for 39 months beyond the trial work period.

For more information about Social Security's work incentives, call either your local Social Security office or the toll-free number previously listed and request a copy of Publication No. 05–10095, *Working While Disabled . . . How Social Security Can Help.*

HOSPITAL AND MEDICAL INSURANCE COVERAGE

Private Medical Insurance

When I left my place of employment in November 1991, I was able to continue my Medical Insurance coverage under COBRA (Continuation of Benefits). This allowed me to continue my coverage with the same group insurance policy for a period of 18 months. It was intended to be a short-term coverage plan until I was able to secure another position. However, I realized in October 1992 that my hopes of securing a new position and a new health insurance policy were rather bleak. I called a number of private health insurance carriers and was told that since I had a terminal disease, my chances of buying health insurance were next to zero. I spoke to my state insurance department and was told that I could buy coverage in a "pool" plan which meant that I could buy coverage at about $1,500 per month, or $18,000 per year.

By this time I had only about three months left on the 18-month COBRA extension. Suffice it to say that I was beginning to panic. I began receiving Social Security disability payments in January 1993 and was advised that I could go on Medicare in two years (January 1995). However, since my COBRA was expected to end in February 1994, I faced the problem of not having any insurance for ten months.

One afternoon while I was reading an article in the American Association of Retired Persons (AARP) magazine, I came across a statement that said that persons under age 65 and receiving Social Security Disability Benefits could extend their COBRA coverage for an additional 11 months. When I called my insurance carrier to inquire how I could apply for this extended coverage, I was told that all I had to do was send them a copy of my Social Security disability award letter. I would then be covered for an additional 11 months.

What Is Medicare?

"If you are like most older Americans covered by Medicare, there are aspects of the federal health insurance program that you find complex and confusing."

No truer words have ever been written by anyone in Washington, D.C., as those found in this quote from the government publication *Guide to Health Insurance for People with Medicare.*[2] As of this writing, existing Medicare and Medicaid programs are under reform pressures that will significantly change or modify the present benefits, deductibles, copayments, and eligibility.

Medicare is a health insurance program administered by the U.S. government for people aged 65 or older, people of any age with permanent kidney failure, and for certain disabled persons under 65. Medicare consists of two parts: Hospital Insurance (Part A) and Medical Insurance (Part B).

Do not confuse Part A and Part B with Plan A or Plan B of the Medigap insurance plans.

Medicare, Part A, is financed through the Social Security tax (FICA) paid by workers and their employers. Part B is optional and is offered to all people when they become eligible for Part A. The premium for Part B is deducted automatically from an individual's monthly Social Security check. (Currently, the 1995 monthly premium is $46.10). Although it is not required that you purchase Part B, considering what private medical health insurance costs, it's a good buy to consider.

Medicare Hospital Insurance Benefits (Part A)

The following is a brief summary of the benefits paid by Medicare for hospital expenses. Several key elements must be defined first before the benefits summary makes any sense to you.

1. Benefit Periods: A benefit period is defined as a period of time beginning when a participant is admitted to a hospital or nursing home that participates in Medicare and ends when the patient has been discharged for more than 60 days. In other words, the benefit period begins when you are admitted to the hospital and ends 60 days after you are discharged.

2. Nonrenewable lifetime reserve days: Each individual has 60 reserve days under Medicare. These lifetime reserve days may be used whenever you are in the hospital for more than 90 consecutive days. Once used, the reserve days are not renewable.

Keeping these two points in mind, the benefit coverage for 1995 follows.

SERVICES	BENEFIT	MEDICARE PAYS	YOU PAY
HOSPITALIZATION Semiprivate room and board, general nursing and other hospital services and supplies.	First 60 Days	All but $716	$716
	61st to 90th day	All but $179 a day	$179 a day
	91st to 150th day	All but $358 a day	$358 a day
	Beyond 150 days	Nothing	All costs
SKILLED NURSING FACILITY CARE You must have been in a hospital for at least 3 days, enter a Medicare-approved facility generally within 30 days after hospital discharge, and meet other program requirements.	First 20 days	100% of approved amount	Nothing
	Additional 80 days	All but $89.50 a day	Up to $89.50 a day
	Beyond 100 days	Nothing	All costs
HOME HEALTH CARE Medically necessary skilled care, home health aide services, medical supplies, etc.	For as long as you meet Medicare requirements for home care benefits.	100% of approved amount; 80% of approved amount for durable medical equipment.	Nothing for services; 20% of approved amount for durable medical equipment.
HOSPICE CARE Pain relief, symptom management and support services for the terminally ill.	For as long as doctor certifies need.	All but limited costs for outpatient drugs and inpatient respite care.	Limited cost sharing for outpatient drugs and inpatient respite care.
BLOOD	Unlimited if medically necessary.	All but first 3 pints per calendar year.	For first 3 pints.

Table 1. Medicare (Part A): Hospital insurance covered services for 1995

From the data shown in Table 1 you can see that there are significant "gaps" in Medicare coverage for inpatient hospital care. The following is a summary of these gaps:

Hospital Coverage Gaps

- You pay $716 deductible on your first admission to a hospital in each benefit period.
- You pay $179 daily "coinsurance" for days 61 through 90.
- There is no coverage beyond 90 days in any benefit period unless you have "lifetime reserve" days available.
- You pay $358 daily coinsurance for each lifetime reserve day used.
- There is no coverage for the first three pints of whole blood or units of packed cells used in each year in connection with covered services. To

the extent that the three-pint blood deductible is met under Part B, it does not have to be met under Part A.

- No coverage for a private hospital room or a private duty nurse is provided unless medically necessary.
- No coverage for personal convenience items is provided, such as a telephone or a television in a hospital room.
- No coverage for care that is not medically necessary or for nonemergency care in a hospital not certified by Medicare.
- No coverage for care received outside the United States and its territories, except under limited circumstances in Canada or Mexico.

Nursing Facility Coverage Gaps

- You pay $89.50 daily coinsurance for days 21 through 100 in each benefit period.
- No coverage beyond 100 days in a benefit period.
- No coverage for care in a nursing home, or in an SNF (Skilled Nursing Facility) not certified by Medicare, or for just custodial care in a Medicare-certified SNF.
- No coverage for three-pint blood deductible.

Gaps in Medicare Home Health Coverage

- No coverage for full-time nursing care.
- No coverage for drugs or meals delivered to your home.
- You pay 20 percent of the Medicare-approved amount for durable medical equipment, plus charges in excess of the approved amount on undersigned claims.
- No coverage for homemaker services that are primarily to assist you in meeting personal care or housekeeping needs.

Gaps in Medicare Hospice Coverage

- You pay limited charges for inpatient respite care and outpatient drugs.
- You pay deductibles and coinsurance amounts when regular Medicare benefits are used for treatment of a condition other than the terminal illness.

Gaps in Medicare Inpatient Psychiatric Hospital Care

- No coverage for care after you have received 190 days of such specialized treatment in your lifetime (even if you have not yet exhausted your
  inpatient hospital coverage).

As you can readily see, while Medicare is a good insurance plan it does not
fully cover the hospital patient and at the very minimum will cost $716 (the
deductible) for each benefit period. As will be covered in a later section, Medigap
insurance becomes a very desirable and usually affordable option.

Medicare Medical Insurance (Part B)

Part B of Medicare is designed to help pay for necessary physician services no
matter where you receive them: at home, at the doctor's office, in a clinic, in a
nursing home, or in a hospital. It also covers related medical services and supplies required in outpatient hospital systems, and X-ray and laboratory tests.
Coverage is also provided for certain ambulance services and for the use of
home medical equipment such as wheelchairs and hospital beds. Part B also
covers physical therapy and occupational therapy for outpatients and inpatients;
however, it does not cover outpatient prescription drugs (although there are
certain exceptions).

Payments to the doctor or therapist are based on a national fee schedule.
Medicare pays 80 percent of the approved amount, and you are responsible for
the balance. Some physicians and medical suppliers will accept assignment of
Medicare claims. This means that they accept the national fee schedule and you
will be responsible only for the 20 percent (after your $100 deductible has been
satisfied). If your doctor does not accept assignment, you are responsible for
paying all permissible charges.

The following table outlines the medical expenses covered under Part B of
Medicare. The data shown is for 1995. Since changes are being contemplated in
the National Health Reform Act, this data should only be used as a guideline.
Similar to Part A, Part B also contains gaps in Medicare coverage. Here is a
brief recap of these gaps:

- You pay a $100 annual deductible.
- Generally, you pay 20 percent coinsurance.
- You pay legally permissible charges in excess of the Medicare-approved
  amount for unassigned claims.
- You pay 50 percent of approved charges for most outpatient mental
  health treatment.

SERVICES	BENEFIT	MEDICARE PAYS	YOU PAY
MEDICAL EXPENSES Physician's services inpatient and outpatient medical and surgical services and supplies, physical and speech therapy, diagnostic tests, durable medical equipment and other services.	Medicare pays for medical services in or out of the hospital.	80% of approved amount (after $100 deductible); 50% of approved charges for most outpatient mental health services	$100 deductible, plus 20% of approved amount and limited charges above approved amount. 50% of approved charges for mental health services.
CLINICAL LABORATORY SERVICES Blood tests, urinalysis, and more.	Unlimited if medically necessary.	Generally 100% of approved amount.	Nothing for services.
HOME HEALTH CARE Medically necessary skilled care, home health aide services, medical supplies, and other services.	For as long as you meet Medicare requirements for home care benefits.	100% of approved amount; 80% of approved amount for durable medical equipment.	Nothing for services; 20% of approved amount for durable medical equipment.
OUTPATIENT HOSPITAL TREATMENT Reasonable and necessary services for the diagnosis or treatment of an illness or injury.	Unlimited if medically necessary.	Medicare payment to hospital based on hospital costs.	20% of billed amount (after $100 deductible).
BLOOD	Unlimited if medically necessary.	80% of approved amount (after $100 deductible and starting with 4th pint).	For first 3 pints plus 20% of approved amount for additional pints (after $100 deductible).

Table 2. Medicare (Part B): Services and benefits

- You pay all charges in excess of Medicare's maximum yearly limit of $900 for independent physical or occupational therapists.

- No coverage is provided for most services that are not reasonable and necessary for the diagnosis or treatment of an illness or injury.

- No coverage is provided for most self-administerable prescription drugs or immunizations, except for pneumococcal, and hepatitis B vaccinations.

- No coverage for routine physical and other screening services, except for mammograms and Pap smears.

- Generally, there is no coverage for dental care or dentures.

- No coverage is provided for acupuncture treatment.

- No coverage is provided for hearing aids or routine hearing loss examinations.

- No coverage is provided for care received outside the United States and its territories, except under limited circumstances in Canada and Mexico.
- No coverage for routine foot care except when a medical condition affecting the lower limbs (such as diabetes) requires care by a medical professional.
- No coverage for services of naturopaths, Christian Science practitioners, immediate relatives, or charges imposed by members of your household.
- No coverage is provided for the first three pints of whole blood or units of packed cells used in each year in connection with covered services. To the extent that the three-pint blood deductible is met under Part A, it does not have to be met under Part B.
- No coverage for routine eye examinations or eyeglasses, except prosthetic lenses, if needed, after cataract surgery.

Medicaid

Because Medicaid is administered differently in different states, it is very difficult to generalize about this medical coverage. Medicaid is an "income qualified" plan, or in other words, a needs-based program administered by a state agency. Basically, it exists to help individuals handle medical costs that they cannot afford. Medicaid operates on combined federal and state funds and serves persons of any age. Many requirements and conditions must be met to obtain aid. To qualify, applicants must have extremely limited income and assets. The set amounts vary from state to state. If an individual's monthly income exceeds his/her basic allowance, that individual may still be eligible for Medicare if he/she incurs medical bills that use up the difference between his/her income and his/her allowance. Usually a social worker or a lawyer, or both, may be required to help cut through multiple layers of red tape.

Medicaid offers basic help coverage, including doctor's office visits, hospitalization, outpatient visits, and medically required nursing home care. As indicated previously, actions by the 104th Congress may significantly modify the benefits of the Medicaid program as well. As of this writing however, Medicaid programs pay all Medicare premiums, deductibles, and copayments for the elderly and disabled with incomes below the federal poverty line. Every state has an advocate organization established primarily to assist individuals in handling and presenting appeals. You, as a patient, have a right to obtain a written decision on your appeal for eligibility. Any denial of Medicaid, whether a delay in coverage, reduction of benefits, or any matter of dispute, can be appealed.

The rules governing Medicaid benefits are very complex and regulations vary from state to state. Here are just some of the very generalized criteria used in determining Medicaid eligibility. The particular details of determining eligibility in your own state should be worked out with expert help familiar with the latest modifications to the "Medicare Catastrophe Coverage Act of 1988."

- A single individual is allowed certain liquid resources, such as cash and bank accounts, while a couple generally is allowed a higher amount. The amount in each case varies from state to state.

- Other resources like an automobile, a home, and some personal household items and clothing are exempt from your total available assets.

- After certain deductions, all net income over a fixed amount is considered to be available to use toward the cost of medical care.

Medigap Insurance

Since Medicare does not offer complete health insurance protection, private insurance can help fill the gaps. In general, it is advisable to purchase the additional protection that private insurance can provide. Medigap insurance is regulated by federal and state laws. Nearly all states, U.S. territories, and the District of Columbia have adopted regulations that limit the number of different Medigap policies to no more than ten standard benefit plans. The plans have letter designations from "A" to "J." Plan A consists of a "basic" benefits package. While states are required to offer up to ten standard Medigap insurance policies, private insurance companies are required to offer only one Medigap plan for disabled persons. In most states, this is the basic Plan A (see table 3).

Accelerated Death Benefit Insurance

I had been on disability for about twelve months when my funds were beginning to run low. Since I was becoming concerned about being able to cover my living as well as my medical expenses, I began looking into Accelerated Death Benefit Insurance options.

Some insurance companies include in their policies an Accelerated Benefit Rider which gives the policyholder the option to receive a portion of his/her policy death benefit proceeds if the insured becomes terminally ill and is not expected to survive more than twelve months. This rider is usually available at no additional cost. In addition, these funds can be used for any reason and give policyholders the ability to meet potential financial burdens caused by their terminal illness without depleting funds that may have been saved for future financial needs. The funds are also available regardless of the policyholder's income level or assets—unlike most government programs.

The amount of the accelerated benefit, which can be paid in a lump sum or in several periodic payments, varies for each policy and company. Generally,

SERVICES	MEDICARE PAYS	PLAN PAYS	YOU PAY
HOSPITALIZATION			
First 60 days	All but $716	$0	$716
61 through 90th day	All but $179 a day	$179 a day	$0
91st day and after:			
While using 60 lifetime reserve days	All but $358 a day	$358 a day	$0
Once lifetime reserve days are used:			
additional 365 days	$0	100%	$0
beyond the additional 365 days	$0	$0	All costs
SKILLED NURSING FACILITY CARE			
First 20 days	All approved amounts	$0	$0
21st through 100th day	All but $89.50 a day	$0	To $89.50 a day
101st day and after	$0	$0	All costs
BLOOD			
First Three Pints	$0	3 pints	$0
Additional Amounts	100%	$0	$0
HOSPICE CARE	All but very limited coinsurance for outpatient drugs and inpatient respite care	$0	Balance

Table 3.   Medicare hospital services per benefit period

SERVICES	MEDICARE PAYS	PLAN PAYS	YOU PAY
MEDICAL EXPENSES			
First $100 of Medicare approved amounts	$0	All costs	$100
Remainder of Medicare approved amounts	80%	20%	$0
Part B Excess Charges	$0	$20	All costs
BLOOD			
First 3 pints	$0	All costs	$0
Next $100 of Medicare approved amounts	$0	$0	$100
Remainder of Medicare approved amounts	$80	20%	$0
CLINICAL LABORATORY SERVICES	100%	$0	$0

Table 4.   Medicare medical services per calendar year

however, the accelerated benefit payment will be more than can be obtained through a policy loan or surrender. To ensure that a portion of the death benefit remains for the beneficiary, there is usually a maximum amount that can be distributed early. One key factor to be considered here, however, is that the accelerated benefit is taxable. To determine this effect on your personal tax situation, you should

SERVICES	MEDICARE PAYS	PLAN PAYS	YOU PAY
HOME HEALTH CARE MEDICARE APPROVED SERVICES			
Medically necessary skilled care services and medical supplies	100%	$0	$0
Durable Medical equipment			
First $100 of Medicare approved amounts	$0	$0	$100
Remainder of Medicare approved amounts	80%	20%	$0

Table 5. Medicare home health care approved services.

review the plan with your tax advisor. By splitting up the distribution of payments over two tax years, the impact of the tax requirement will be reduced.

Remember, in order to be eligible for accelerated benefits, your doctor needs to attest to the fact that you have a terminal illness or disease that will result in death within 12 months or less. If, however, the insured lives beyond the 12-month expectancy, the accelerated benefit payment does not need to be repaid.

Federal Benefits for Veterans

Eligibility for most VA benefits is based on the veteran's condition when discharged from active military service. Active service means full-time service as a member of the armed forces or as a commissioned officer of several public-service organizations such as the Public Health Service. The Defense Department issues each veteran a military discharge form, DD 214. This form, as well as a certified copy of your marriage license (if married), is required when filing for VA benefits for the first time.

Certain VA benefits and medical care require wartime service. Disability pensions for nonmilitary-connected disabilities require that at least one day of your active military service was served during a period of war. As specified by law, the VA recognizes the following war periods:

Mexican Border Period	May 9, 1916, through April 5, 1917
World War I	April 6, 1917, through November 11, 1918
World War II	December 7, 1941, through December 31, 1946
Korean Conflict	June 27, 1950, through January 31, 1955
Vietnam Era	August 5, 1964, through May 7, 1975
Persian Gulf War	August 2, 1990, through a date to be set by law or by a Presidential Proclamation

Veterans with service-connected disabilities more than likely have already begun to receive VA benefits and are aware of the multiple disability benefits packages available from the VA. I will therefore skip to those veterans who have become disabled for reasons neither traceable to military service nor to willful misconduct. These veterans are eligible for support if they have limited income and have had 90 days or more of active duty with at least one day of which was during a period of war listed previously. If you are permanently and totally disabled, payments are made to bring your total income, including other retirement income or Social Security income, to an established support level as shown in the following table. According to the 1994 Improved Pension program,[3] the following maximum annual rates are generally paid monthly to veterans. These amounts may be reduced depending on the amount of the annual income of the veteran and the income of his/her spouse or dependent children.

- Veteran without dependent spouse or child $7,818
- Veteran with one dependent spouse or child $10,240
- Veteran in need of regular aid and attendance with no dependents $12,504
- Veteran in need of regular aid and attendance with one dependent $14,927
- Veteran permanently housebound with no dependents $9,556
- Veteran permanently housebound with one dependent $11,977
- Two veterans married to one another $10,240
- Veteran of World War I and Mexican Border Period, add to the applicable annual rate $1,769
- Increase for each additional dependent child $1,330

One feature of VA benefits that should be carefully examined is that a veteran who is a patient in a nursing home, or is in need of regular aid and attendance of another person, or is permanently housebound may be entitled to additional benefits. Therefore, make sure that you are properly classified by your VA regional office. Keep in mind that applicants of VA benefits have the right to appeal determinations made by a VA regional office or by a medical center.

FEDERAL, STATE, AND COMMUNITY SERVICES

It is impossible to cover all federal, state and local community programs that offer emergency-type funding and services. Funds are made available to state agencies each year through the Older Americans Act and are generally available to anyone over the age of 60. Your local Social Security office can provide information as to what organizations are available in your immediate area. Some of these organizations include Meals on Wheels and adult day-care centers. Your local clergy or social worker can also help you locate services to help you cope with day-to-day problems. Also consult volunteer health organizations, such as the Arthritis Foundation. These organizations usually have listings of services available in any community.

General Help

MORTGAGE HOLDERS

When it became evident that my condition was not going to improve, my wife and I needed to sort out our entire financial situation.

Deferred Principal Payments

One of the first items on our agenda was how we were going to pay the mortgage on our house. We were on a variable-rate mortgage plan and were already paying the lowest rate possible. This fact prevented us from refinancing our mortgage to obtain a lower monthly payment.

I went to my lending officer and explained to him my situation. I told him of my diagnosis, and to my surprise, he told me that his father had died from ALS. He was very sympathetic to our problem and suggested that the bank defer some of our principal payments for a period of time. While this did not generate enormous savings, it did buy us a bit of time.

The point that I wish to make with this example is that before your lender comes after you for late payments, go to your lender first and explain your situation. You will find that lenders are more than willing to help you work out a financial problem before you become delinquent on your payments.

Reverse Mortgages

The reverse mortgage is a relatively new type of loan that doesn't need to be repaid until the borrower either sells the house or dies. This loan simply works backwards or in "reverse." Based on the equity on your home, you can arrange for fixed monthly payments to you or a fixed line of credit from which you can draw varying amounts depending solely on your needs. When the house is sold, either upon the death of the borrower or at the borrower's discretion, the loan is repaid along with accrued interest from the proceeds of the sale.

Reverse mortgages are available in 47 states (Alaska, South Dakota, and

Texas being the exceptions). The concept of the reverse mortgage has been around for a while but has not been widely used or available until the Federal Housing Administration developed its own plan. The involvement of the FHA brought not only strict rules, rates, and fees, but also added security of the government's loan guarantee to lenders. Essentially, there are three types of plans that are offered by both FHA-backed loans and loans from private lenders:

- **Term plan.** This plan pays a fixed monthly payment for a fixed period of time.

- **Tenure plan.** This plan guarantees a fixed monthly amount for as long as you live in your house. Since the lender cannot be sure how long you are going to live, the monthly amount is much smaller than under the term plan.

- **Line of credit plan.** Operates much like any typical home equity plan whereby you can draw cash at any time. The major differences, however, are that there are no monthly principal and interest repayments.

To qualify for the reverse mortgage loan, you only need to have equity in your home. Your age, however, is also important because the older you are, the more you can borrow from your equity. If you still owe on a mortgage or another debt secured by your home, you must pay it off before obtaining a reverse mortgage.

Reverse mortgages do not require that you transfer ownership to a lender. The lender has no claim on assets other than what the house is worth when it is sold. If you borrowed more than the proceeds cover, the lender cannot ask your heirs to make up the difference.

FHA offers free counseling through local nonprofit and public agencies. For additional information regarding reverse mortgages, contact the following:

AARP Home Equity Information Center EE0756
601 E Street NW
Washington, DC 20049

AARP Home Equity Conversion Information Kit (D15601)
601 E Street NW
Washington, DC 20049

In addition, *Your New Retirement Nest Egg: A Consumer Guide to the New Reverse Mortgages* (Ken Scholen, National Center for Home Equity Conversion, 1995) discusses reverse mortgages, cash benefits, total loan costs, and left-over equity. The following is a sample schedule of loans and monthly payments based on the data from this guide.

The Consumer Credit Counseling, Inc. is a nationwide organization whose

HOME VALUE	BORROWER'S AGE	LUMP SUM OR CREDIT LINE	MONTHLY PAYMENT* (TENURE)
$50,000	65	$ 9,933	$ 81
	70	13,203	110
	75	16,916	147
	80	21,147	196
	85	25,587	265
	90	30,103	386
$100,000	65	25,333	207
	70	31,803	265
	75	39,116	339
	80	47,397	438
	85	55,987	580
	90	64,553	829
$150,000	65	40,733	332
	70	50,403	420
	75	61,316	532
	80	73,647	681
	85	86,387	895
	90	99,003	1,271

* Assumptions: 9% expected interest rate, $1,800 origination fee, 2% mortgage interest premium, $25 monthly servicing fee, and closing costs totaling $1,000 on a $50,000 home, $1,400 on a $100,000 home, and $1,800 on a $150,000 home.

Table 6.   Cash benefits from an FHA-insured reverse mortgage[4]

sole purpose is to assist individuals and their families in dealing with potential credit problems. When it became obvious that I needed help in paying my ever-growing debt, I called the CCC Organization and made an appointment to meet with a counselor. I was told to gather records of all of my fixed and variable monthly expenses and to come to the office for a one-hour planning session.

The counselor and I constructed a monthly budget based on what limited income I had and what assets I could make available for expense payments. We worked out a realistic approach to fixed payments such as mortgages, taxes, and credit card debt. On the basis of this realistic budget, the Consumer Credit counselor offered to call my various creditors and arrange for reduced monthly payments that were within my ability to pay.

THE AMERICANS WITH DISABILITIES ACT

If you build it, they will come.

—from the movie *Field of Dreams*

Shortly after I obtained my powerchair, my wife and I made dinner reservations at a very well-known restaurant/inn. When we arrived at the restaurant, we discovered that there was no handicap parking available and that the main entrance to the restaurant consisted of a flight of six steps. We were told that we could enter the restaurant from the parking lot, which was in the rear of the inn. I finally found a spot at the rear of the unpaved parking lot to unload my powerchair. Using full power on my chair, I bounced across the rough gravel surface to a rear service entrance. From there I traveled through a service corridor of the inn and through a retail shop. When we finally arrived at the restaurant, we were assigned a table close to the rear service entrance door because of the congested placement of the tables and chairs. To top off the evening, we ended up being treated quite shoddily by the servers.

On July 26, 1990, President Bush signed the Americans with Disabilities Act (ADA). This act is a federal law which provides persons with disabilities protection from discrimination in areas of employment, public accommodation, state and local government services, telecommunications, and transportation. This law protects the disabled against discrimination in the same manner as the laws that protect individuals from being discriminated against on the basis of race, color, national origin, sex, and religion.

In brief, this law states that persons with disabilities should be treated the same as persons without disabilities. A person with a disability ought to be able to enter a restaurant, for example, in the same manner as a person without a disability. The ADA defines a person with a disability as someone who:

1. Has a physical or mental impairment which limits one or more major life activities (such as working, learning, walking, seeing, etc.); or

2. Has a record of having had such an impairment; or

3. Who is seen or regarded as having such an impairment.

An individual with a hidden disability, such as a learning disability, or an individual who is perceived to be disabled even if he/she is not (for example, someone who has a disfigured face or severe scars) must also be treated in the same manner as a person without a disability.

The Americans with Disabilities Act defines a place of public accommodation as a "private entity which serves the public." This includes hotels, motels, restaurants, physicians' offices, places of recreation and education, barbershops, beauty salons, office buildings, and similar places of business. In regard to access to these places of public accommodation, all new construction must be fully accessible and usable to people with disabilities. Religious facilities and certain private clubs are not considered places of public accommodation if their activities are limited to members only.

Since my awful restaurant experience, I educated myself more about the law and its provisions, and as a result I was able to file a complaint form. Once completed, the written complaint form should be sent to:

Department of Justice
Civil Rights Division
ADA Compliance Office, Post Office Box 66118
Washington, DC 20035-6118
(202) 514-0301 or TDD (202) 514-0383

The Americans with Disabilities Act is only a beginning. Although the law has been in effect for over two years as of this writing, there are still thousands of places of public accommodation that I cannot enter. For example, in the early part of 1994, I visited my family physician's office and discovered that they were reconstructing the entrance to the building. Although wheelchair users were now able to open the entrance doors by simply pressing a button from the outside, no such button existed inside the building. Therefore wheelchair users could only enter the building. After complaining to the contractor of the building, an inside button was finally installed.

In my lifetime, I would like to see all public accommodation entities comply with the Americans with Disabilities Act. I had to essentially stop my business activities because of access barriers. The small businesses that I dealt with usually were not equipped to accommodate disabled persons.

When employment discrimination exists, you may file a formal complaint against a business by contacting the Equal Employment Opportunity Commission (EEOC) at the following address:

Equal Employment Opportunity Commission (EEOC)
Tenth Street and Constitution Avenue
Washington, DC 20530
(202) 663-4900, (800) 872-3362, or TDD (800) 800-3302

In addition, a private lawsuit in federal court may be filed.

If discrimination is found, employers may be ordered to place a person with a disability into the job sought. Employers may also be responsible for back pay as well as attorney's fees and costs. In cases of intentional discrimination, an employer may also be forced to pay compensatory and punitive damages.

For more information regarding the Americans with Disabilities Act, refer to the following guide: *Accessibility: It's Yours for the Asking* (D15520). To obtain a copy, write to:

AARP Fulfillment (EE0739)
Post Office Box 22796,
Long Beach, CA 90801-5796

The diagrams and illustrations on the following pages are examples of how specific areas can be made accessible to disabled individuals.

Accessible Doorway

- 32" minimum clear width
- 24" clear space (on pull side)
- Maximum force to open: 5 pounds

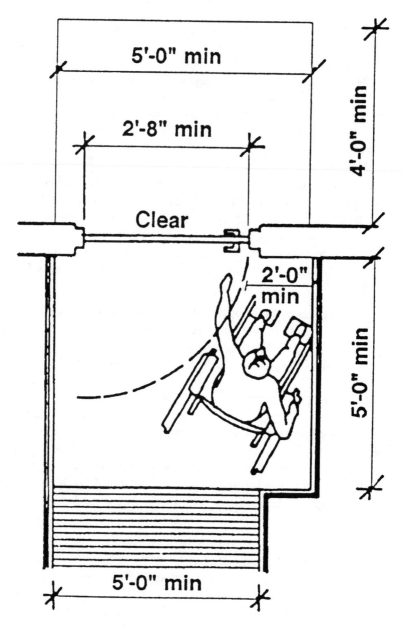

Figure 50. Accessible Doorway

Accessible Parking Space

- Raised Sign: "Handicapped Parking State permit required Violators will be fined."

- Parking Space: 12' minimum width
- Crosshatching: 3' minimum width

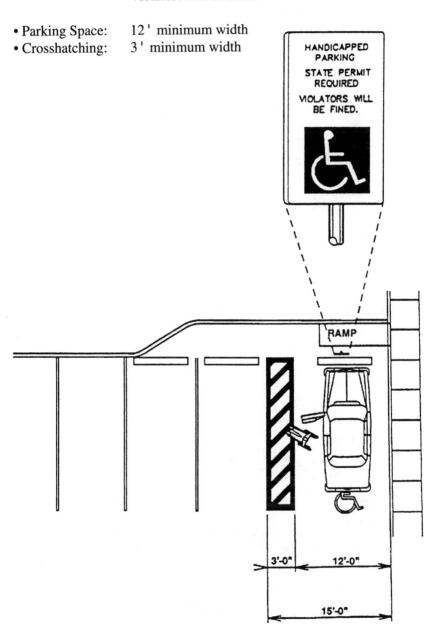

Figure 51. Accessible Parking Space

Curb Cut

- 3' minimum curb width
- 4' minimum walkway width
- 1:12 maximum slope (middle)
- 1:10 maximum slope (sides)
- Lip must be flush with street

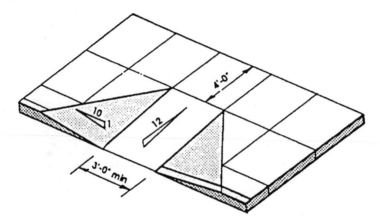

Water Fountain

- Working parts at 27"–36" height

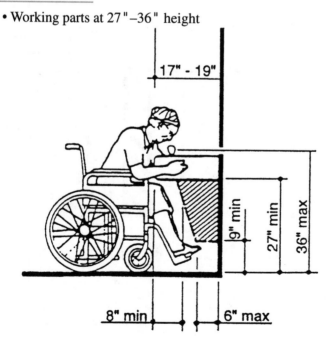

Figure 52. Curb Cut and Water Fountain

Ramp

- Minimum landing length: 60" at top and bottom, and at 30' intervals of ramp
- Minimum clear width: 36"
- Handrails required:
  If rise is greater than 6" or if horizontal projection is greater than 72"

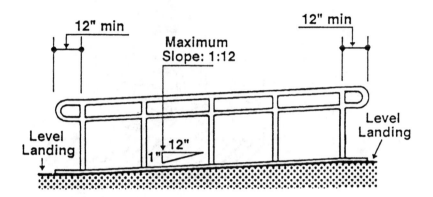

Cane Range for Detecting Objects

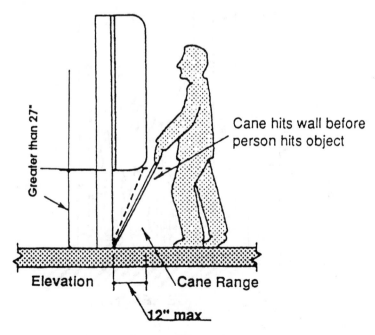

Figure 53. Ramp and Cane Range of Detection

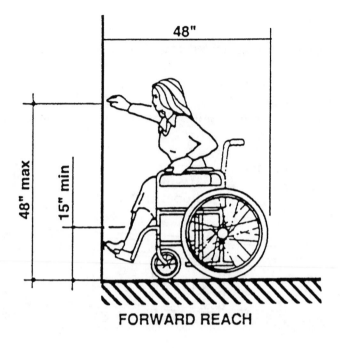

FORWARD REACH

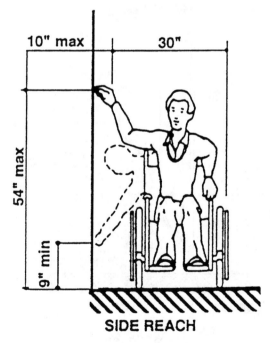

SIDE REACH

Figure 54. Reach Limits

Telephone

- All working parts no higher than 48"
- Minimum clear floor space: 30" x 48"

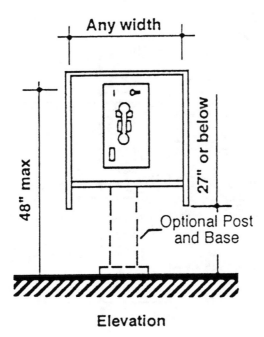

Elevation

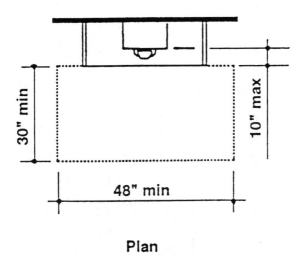

Plan

Figure 55. Accessible Telephone

Lavatory

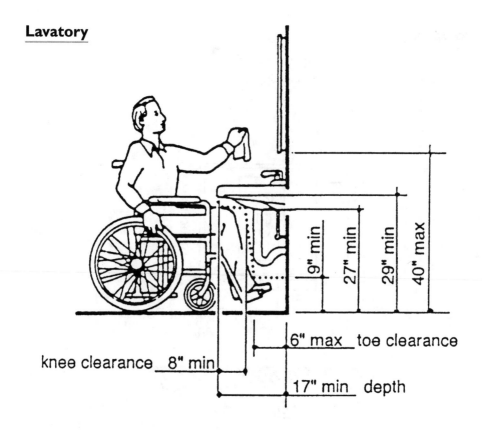

9" min

27" min

29" min

40" max

6" max   toe clearance

knee clearance   8" min

17" min   depth

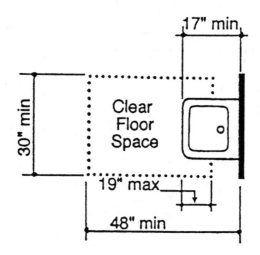

17" min

30" min

Clear
Floor
Space

19" max

48" min

Figure 56.   Lavatory

Toilet Stalls

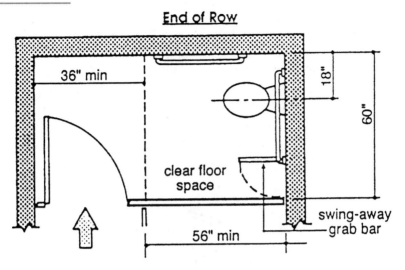

Figure 59. Toilet Stalls

Elevator

- Call buttons: centered at 42" height
- Hall lanterns: minimum 72" height
- Minimum door width: 36"
- Raised and braille numbers on door jambs: 60" height
- Interior control buttons: braille and raised numbers maximum 48" height (front approach)

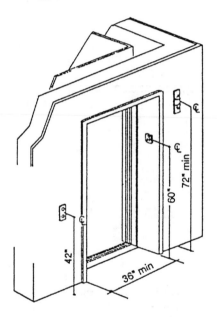

Control panel with tactile markings

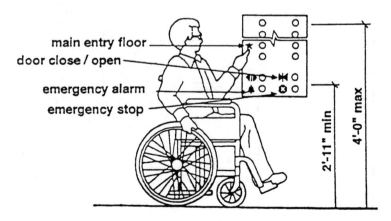

main entry floor
door close / open
emergency alarm
emergency stop

Figure 58. Elevator

And in Conclusion

The ultimate goal of this book is to help you to become your own advocate. In the process you will be able to take charge of your life if faced with a traumatic illness or disability.

Part IV Notes

1. U.S. Department of Health and Human Services, *Disability* (Social Security Administration, Publication No. 05–10029).

2. *Guide to Health Insurance for People with Medicare.* (Developed jointly by the National Association of Insurance Commissioners and the Health Care Financing Administration of the U.S. Department of Health and Human Services, Publication No. HCFA–02110, 1994).

3. "Federal Benefits for Veterans and Dependents, 1994 Edition" (Department of Veterans Affairs, VA Pamphlet 80-94–1, 1994).

4. Table 6 adapted from *Your New Retirement Nest Egg: A Consumer Guide to the New Reverse Mortgages* (National Center for Home Equity Conversion, 1995).

Index